Hazards in Hospital Care

Shizuko Y. Fagerhaugh
Anselm Strauss
Barbara Suczek
Carolyn L. Wiener

Hazards in Hospital Care

Ensuring Patient Safety

 Jossey-Bass Publishers
San Francisco • London • 1987

HAZARDS IN HOSPITAL CARE
Ensuring Patient Safety
by Shizuko Y. Fagerhaugh, Anselm Strauss, Barbara Suczek, and
Carolyn L. Wiener

Copyright © 1987 by: Jossey-Bass Inc., Publishers
433 California Street
San Francisco, California 94104
&
Jossey-Bass Limited
28 Banner Street
London EC1Y 8QE

Library of Congress Cataloging-in-Publication Data

Hazards in hospital care.

(A Joint publication in the Jossey-Bass health
series and the Jossey-Bass social and behavioral
science series)
Bibliography: p.
Includes index.
1. Hospitals—Safety measures. 2. Medical errors—
Prevention. I. Fagerhaugh, Shizuko Y. II. Series:
Jossey-Bass social and behavioral science series.
[DNLM: 1. Accident Prevention. 2. Hospital Administra-
tion. 3. Patients. 4. Quality Assurance, Health Care.
WX 185 H428]
RA969.9.H39 1987   362.1′1   87-45509
ISBN 1-55542-073-7 (alk. paper)

Manufactured in the United States of America

The paper in this book meets the guidelines for
permanence and durability of the Committee on
Production Guidelines for Book Longevity of the
Council on Library Resources.

JACKET DESIGN BY WILLI BAUM

FIRST EDITION

Code 8748

A joint publication in
The Jossey-Bass Health Series
and
The Jossey-Bass
Social and Behavioral Science Series

Contents

Preface

The hospital is virtually the only type of organization that is quite literally organized around the issue of safety: specifically, the clinical safety of patients. Paradoxically, the hospital's mission centers around decreasing the hazards of illness to people who enter already endangered. This is done largely through an armamentarium of technical means (drugs, equipment, procedures, surgeries) and the specific knowledge associated with those means. At the same time, this sophisticated and rapidly changing technology can pose great hazards in its specific use. Modern medical and nursing care consists of interventions into the natural course of a disease. All interventions are potentially risky, and medical judgment consists—whether implicitly or explicitly—of weighing the risks of various alternative interventions against the anticipated natural course of a given illness.

How do those who work in hospitals organize their individual and collective work as they attempt to ensure the safety of patients? This and a number of related questions are at the heart of this book: How are decisions about safety and hazards made? How are hazards foreseen, avoided, managed, or dealt with when misjudged or when errors have been made? What part do organizational arrangements and strategies play in helping to maximize clinical safety and to minimize the hazards to it? Under what conditions do the organizational arrangements/strategies or the personnel fail in assuring safety, and why? How can social scientists contribute to improving the safety in patient care?

After observing a number of hospital wards and interviewing people there, and having identified clinical safety as a major
aim for staff members but also a critical problem for them, we
decided to address these kinds of questions. We developed a
theoretical formulation that emphasizes three important and interrelated foci: (1) the hospital as an organization, (2) interaction
among the personnel and between the personnel and the patients,
and (3) chronic illnesses, which are the predominant causes of
patient hospitalization.

Because we are sociologists, though one of us is also a
nurse, we bring a sociological perspective to the safety arena
and to the wards themselves. During our research, we became
convinced that problems of safety in hospitals could not be solved
without taking the organizational aspects of hospitals into account as well as the accompanying interactional dynamics. In
the larger research study, of which this book is a product, we
had already grasped that a combination of evolving medical
technology and the changed character of illness (chronic illnesses
are now prevalent in developed countries) had profoundly altered
the structure of the hospital and the work of its personnel (Strauss,
Fagerhaugh, Suczek, and Wiener, 1985). To the best of our
knowledge, no other approach to clinical safety looks at it as
we shall do in this book.

In writing *Hazards in Hospital Care*, we hope that several
different audiences will profit from reading it. These include
practitioners who are quite literally at the bedside—nurses,
physicians, social workers, various technicians—as well as personnel in the supporting services—hospital administrators, especially nursing administrators and supervisors, pharmacists,
bioengineers, and safety engineers. We hope, too, that people
who are involved with the area of health policy—specifically,
legislators, governmental administrators, and researchers—will
read what we have written. We have also written for social scientists, especially our colleagues in medical sociology and in the
sociology of work/professions. Perhaps it is not too presumptu-
ous to hope that some laypeople might be enlightened by what
lies between the covers of this book. They will then know better
how hard and carefully hospital personnel work at maximizing

their chances for safe care; after all, patients usually enter the hospital in a more or less hazardous condition but leave in an improved condition. They will also know something of why the personnel sometimes fail in this effort. Practitioners should find a number of discussions that shed light on their difficulties and that encourage them to think in more organizational and more negotiatory/communicative terms about safety problems. Policy-makers might begin to have second thoughts about what is involved in quality care and how an industrial model of the "health industry" may not fit, and indeed may somewhat hinder, giving the best patient care. The social scientists in our anticipated audience will get a picture of aspects of both the acute care hospital and hospital work that is not yet in their literature. They will find a further elaboration of the substantive theory developed in our previous book.

Chapter One discusses the difficulties of assuring patients' safety, given the nature of chronic illness and the impact of rapidly evolving medical technology on the work and organization of hospitals. Related to both are various debates over complex issues, involving legal questions, moral questions, problems of dehumanization and equity, and also technical questions concerning technological assessment and risk assessment. Of course, one issue that is especially prominent today is cost containment. Given the numbers and types of participants arguing over and acting on these issues, augmented by the rise of the patients' rights movement, we can expect the management of clinical safety to be directly or indirectly affected. And indeed it is.

In Chapter Two we present a theoretical framework organized around the concept of illness trajectory. This framework will be elaborated in the chapters that follow. Our discussion touches on a set of interrelated safety work processes (assessing, monitoring, preventing, and rectifying hazards). These arise from many sources—patient behavior (the patient as a person), the clinical interventions, the staff, the environment, and organizational arrangement—and pertain to the management of the various types of potential risk (clinical, identity, and comfort). This management is at the level of the overall trajectory and the task. That is, the trajectory formulation analyzes safety work done over the entire course of an illness in terms of the changing contingencies that alter the safety work processes and types of hazard concerns. Since safety work occurs within a complex organizational/interactional context, the trajectory formulation takes into account the professionals' concerns about hazards bearing on their own identities (legal, economic, interactional, moral-ethical), which in turn shape how clinical safety is managed. Our framework also includes a focus on the immense amount of safety work engaged in by patients and kin. A case study in this chapter is included to illustrate these points.

In Chapter Three we examine the complexity of controlling the various medical/technical hazards related to diagnosis, palliation, and treatment of diseases. The complicated relationships of the many sources of hazard and the consequence for safety work are then analyzed. Because hospitals are dense with machines, various machine-related hazards are also noted. In addition, a conditional matrix of the dimensions of hazards and their sources is suggested as a means for understanding more clearly the complexity of clinical safety work as well as its constantly changing character as a given illness evolves.

The discussion in Chapter Four covers the four work processes for ensuring safety: preventing, monitoring, assessing, and rectifying hazards. A notable feature of each is the many types and levels of workers who are involved in attempting to control the numerous hazards. Because their work overlaps, constant negotiation is necessary so that they can align their respective tasks. Safety work processes can be disrupted because the personnel may feel that controlling certain hazards takes priority over controlling others, and they may also vary in which specific risk they are weighing and balancing. Another matrix is presented that deals with differences among staff, patient, and family concerning which risks are being balanced. The matrix should help staff to identify the sources of conflict concerning risk assessments. Also discussed is how important it is to develop effective means of communication about a patient's status and prescribed care, because of the multiplicity of care givers who may have differing priorities.

Chapter Five is devoted to an examination of the management of clinical errors, since errors made by staff can have fateful consequences for patients, staff, and the hospital itself. Difficulties that affect error management are discussed, including the sophistication of technologies, combined with the problematic character of some chronic illnesses and the complex types and sources of human error. We pay particular attention to the interactional difficulties involved in giving care and their relevance for staff's attempts to find solutions when errors are made.

Chapter Six addresses the patient's contributions to safety work, explaining why staff should recognize it explicitly and promote further participation in it. Examples are given of patients' and families' safety work. And various difficulties surrounding ''informed consent,'' conflict over risk assessment, and other exchanges of information involving patients and staff are discussed.

Chapter Seven discusses the relationship between caring and comfort work, and its relevance to clinical safety. We make the point that comfort work is essential for clinical safety and constitutes an important type of safety work in and of itself. The assessment and remedying of discomforts, nurses' philosophies and actions with regard to comfort care, and the consequences of competition between medical-nursing work and comfort work are explored. ''Sentimental work,'' which includes enhancement of patient trust and composure, is also described. We discuss the need to make this kind of work explicit and institutionally accountable in order to ensure its contribution to maximum clinical safety. We also explain the difficulties of this type of work and its importance in preventing the dehumanization of care.

In Chapter Eight, we note the organizational tactics that are designed to maximize clinical safety. These involve articulation of the many interrelated types of work, clusters of tasks, and work processes that are involved in attempts to assure maximal clinical safety. The hospital's need to remain financially solvent in the face of current cutbacks in governmental financial assistance and governmental regulations has implications for safety work. We discuss these and the significance of patients', clinicians', and administrators' recognition that safety is of primary importance. Various organizational mechanisms for quality assurance and risk management are also described, along with their consequences for clinical safety.

In the final chapter, we draw some general implications and a few additional clinical implications from the materials presented in the body of the book. We emphasize the need for a much more integrated approach to managing clinical safety and discuss the need to improve accountability for safety activities and to understand the kinds of phenomena presented in this book. We also point out that efforts to improve safety accountability will have to take into consideration such barriers as competition among and disparate points of view of those involved. We come around again to a recurrent theme in this book: the need for shared power among hospital personnel and willingness on their parts to discuss safety issues openly among themselves and with the general public. We offer policy suggestions that center on the complex and demanding processes involved in managing chronic illness and the need to see chronic illness in terms of the inevitable phases that require attention to safety issues in and outside of the hospital. There is also a brief methodological appendix.

You can see that these chapters are densely packed with descriptive details and with interpretations of them. To summarize these contents in a few lines is not an easy task. In general, however, we would say this: our approach to clinical safety issues is an organizational one and includes a focus on the interaction of health personnel and patients. This approach takes into account both the prevalence of chronic illness and the explosion of medical technology to manage these illnesses. It carefully links major safety work processes (preventing, monitoring, assessing, and rectifying) with courses of illness, and it suggests the need for an overall focus by staff members on their safety management that is explicit, openly discussed, and organizational in emphasis.

For support of the research on which much of this book is based, we are greatly indebted to the Health Resources Administration, Bureau of Manpower, United States Public Health

Service, Division of Nursing, Grant #NU-00598. We are indebted to the staffs of the following Bay Area hospitals where we did extensive fieldwork: Alta Bates, Herrick, Letterman, Mt. Zion, Presbyterian, Stanford, and University of California, and to St. Bartholomew, London, with special thanks to Helen Collyers.

Our thanks also for their various contributions to this book—for data, ideas, reading of the draft manuscript—go to Diane Beeson, University of California, San Francisco; Robert Broadhead, University of Connecticut, Storrs, Connecticut; the late Rue Bucher, Department of Sociology, University of Illinois, Chicago; Wolfram Fischer, University of Muenster, West Germany; Berenice Fisher, New York University, New York City; Elihu Gerson, Tremont Research Institute, San Francisco, California; Roberta Lessor, School of Nursing, University of California, San Francisco; Evelyn Peterson, School of Nursing, University of South Dakota; Fritz Schuetze, University of Kassel, West Germany; Leigh Star, Department of Social and Behavioral Sciences, University of California, San Francisco, and Tremont Research Institute, San Francisco; Steven Wallace, Department of Social and Behavioral Sciences, University of California, San Francisco; Irma Zuckermann, Department of Social and Behavioral Sciences, University of California, San Francisco. We are especially grateful to Barney Glaser for his valuable consultation on the research and to Rue Bucher for her careful reading, editing, and general commentary on the next-to-final draft. Finally, our very special thanks go to Sally Maeth for her patient and persistent secretarial assistance and to the Department of Social and Behavioral Sciences, UCSF, which contributed additional secretarial funding after our grant money ran out.

San Francisco, California   Shizuko Y. Fagerhaugh
August 1987   Anselm Strauss
                                     Barbara Suczek
                                     Carolyn L. Wiener

The Authors

Shizuko Y. Fagerhaugh is visiting lecturer and research nurse in the Department of Social and Behavioral Sciences in the School of Nursing, University of California, San Francisco. She received her B.S. degree in nursing (1947) from Hamline University, St. Paul, Minnesota, her M.A. degree in nursing (1962) from San Francisco State University, and her D.N.Sc. degree (1972) from the University of California, San Francisco. Her main research activities have been related to social problems and issues in chronic illness care. Her writings include *The Politics of Pain Management: Staff-Patient Interactions* (1977, with Anselm Strauss), *Chronic Illness and the Quality of Life* (1984, with Anselm Strauss and others), and *The Social Organization of Medical Work* (1985, with the authors of this book).

Anselm Strauss is professor emeritus of sociology, University of California, San Francisco. He received his B.S. degree in biology (1939) from the University of Virginia, and his M.A. and Ph.D. degrees in sociology (1942 and 1945) from the University of Chicago.

Strauss's main research activities have been in medical sociology and in the sociology of work/professions. His research program in medical sociology goes back over two decades and includes studies on dying in hospitals, the management of pain in hospitals, the impact of medical technology on the care of hospitalized patients, and the problems of living with chronic illness. In 1981 he received the Distinguished Medical Sociologist of the Year award from the Medical Sociology section of the American Sociological Association. He received the Cooley Award (1980) and the Mead Award (1985) from the Society for the Study of Symbolic Interaction and was named the 30th Annual Research Scholar of the Year at the University of California, San Francisco (1987). Strauss is a fellow of the American Association for the Advancement of Science (1980). His publications include *Psychiatric Ideologies and Institutions* (1964, with others), *Awareness of Dying* (1965, with B. Glaser), *The Discovery of Grounded Theory* (1967, with B. Glaser), *Time for Dying* (1968, with B. Glaser), *The Politics of Pain Management* (1977, with S. Fagerhaugh), *The Social Organization of Medical Work* (1985, with others), and *Qualitative Analysis* (1987).

He has been a visiting professor at the University of Cambridge (England), the University of Paris, the University of Manchester, the University of Constance, the University of Adelaide, and the University of Hagen.

Barbara Suczek is a lecturer in sociology and gerontology at San Francisco State University. She received her B.A. degree in 1967 from the University of California, Berkeley, and her M.A. and Ph.D. degrees in sociology (1972 and 1977) from the University of California, San Francisco.

Carolyn L. Wiener is a research sociologist in the Department of Physiological Nursing at the University of California, San Francisco, where she is also a visiting lecturer in the Department of Social and Behavioral Sciences and is affiliated with the Institute for Health and Aging. She received her B.A. degree in interdisciplinary social science (1972) from San Francisco State University, and her M.A. and Ph.D. degrees in sociology (1975 and 1978) from the University of California, San Francisco. Her publications include *The Politics of Alcoholism (1981)* and *The Social Organization of Medical Work* (1985, with Strauss, Fagerhaugh and Suczek). She is currently project director of a study on the treatment of acute illness in nursing homes.

Hazards in Hospital Care

1

∽⌒∽⌒∽⌒∽⌒∽⌒∽⌒∽⌒∽⌒∽⌒∽⌒∽⌒∽⌒∽⌒∽⌒∽⌒∽

Medical Technology
and the Difficulties
of Ensuring Safe Care

The now popular term *technological imperative* was originally used by Fuchs (1968) to suggest that the addition of any new technology generates an increase in further use—whether necessary or not—by its very existence, and this in turn generates still more technology. For understanding what happens in hospitals, we have coined a parallel term, the *errorless imperative*—the drive to eliminate error from work that is associated with medical technology.

Medical machinery, for example, is continually being made more sophisticated for doing work that humans cannot do (split-second monitoring) and for protecting against human error and machine failure (back-up mechanisms and danger alarms). However, these increasingly sophisticated machines require that staffs learn new skills for correctly operating them. Also, machines wear down, and back-up systems break down. So, paradoxically, this technology can increase the chances of danger as well as decrease them. Meanwhile, patients are not inanimate objects so they, too, can be sources of contributory error leading to danger. All of these factors necessitate the learning of new skills and the organizing of institutional resources for servicing and maintaining the equipment, in order to prevent or correct errors. Besides the medical machinery, there are other technologies that involve drugs, devices, and procedures.

Although usually beneficial, these, too, are potentially hazardous. This possibility, when combined with hospital staffs' growing concern with the legal risk of negligence, results in the com-
pelling drive for keeping errors to a minimum.

Technological imperative has led, then, to errorless imperative, which in turn has led to a need for a *safety technology*.
This third term refers both to the work arrangements (division
of labor and the coordination of work tasks) among the many
hospital personnel and the organizational arrangements necessary for guarding against and managing the inevitable hazards
attending the use of technologies. Of course, hospitals have
always instituted measures to control hazards, but the importance of organized safety measures looms very large in today's
highly technologized hospitals. Hospital staffs are organized to
diagnose, treat, and palliate disease, but always in the context
of "do no harm to the patient."

This chapter contains an overview of the impact of medical
technology on patient care, on the work of health workers, on
health professionals and occupations, and on hospital organization. The discussion will also note the complexly interrelated
clinical, social, economic, and ethical dilemmas generated by
medical technology and the consequent difficulties health workers
face in assuring safe patient care.

We wish at this point to address frankly a feature of our
book that may otherwise be upsetting to some readers. Because
the book focuses on safety issues attending patient care, the
various types of errors and mistakes made by health workers
must be discussed carefully and fully. Practitioners who are faced
with doing no harm to the patient under highly uncertain medical
situations and who must contend with many difficult dilemmas
may at times feel our criticism is unfair. However, we as researchers were struck by how well health practitioners—in spite of the
difficult and complex conditions of their work situations in which
many things could go wrong—managed the care so that most
patients experienced no major mishaps. Our intent is not at all
to place blame but to point to the centrality of safety activities
and issues in hospitals today. Indeed, it is safe to say that hospitals are primarily organized around these activities and issues.

Our intent is to describe these so that they may be better understood. A deeper understanding of them should surely lead to an improved safety technology.

For purposes of clarity, we shall make more explicit what is meant by medical technology and make important conceptual distinctions among hazard, danger and risk. The term *medical technology* will be used here in a broad sense as doing something that results in the modification of products, services, and processes. Technology involves "a self-conscious organized means of affecting the physical and social environment—objected and transmitted to others" (Frekin, 1969, p. 11). Thus, medical technology includes both hardware (equipment and facilities) and software (knowledge, skills, and social organization).

In many current writings, hazard, danger, and risk are used synonymously. We must distinguish carefully among them to avoid that confusion here, for they will be central terms in this book. *Danger* will refer to injury, loss, pain, or other threat from an illness itself, or contingencies not dependent on human (professional or patient) action. *Risk,* on the other hand, will refer to injury, loss, pain, or other threat that derives from doing something or not doing something (treatment, drugs, physical or mechanical action, and so on), whether by professionals or patients. In short, risk here means, as commonly used in medical parlance, "taking a calculated risk"—it involves weighing the possible negative consequences resulting from a given action or "intervention" in trying to affect the course of a patient's illness. *Hazard* will be the most general term, standing for both danger (from illness) and risk (from interventions).

To comprehend technology-related hazards management properly in the acute care hospital, it is necessary to understand certain features of the larger context within which the management occurs. During the 1940s and 1950s, as a consequence of tremendous medical technological advances made in diagnosing and treating diseases, societal optimism about medicine blossomed: medical science could eventually control disease. This optimism was supported by generous governmental financing of medical research and development. In those decades the discovery of new miracle drugs, sulfonamides, penicillin and other antibiotics, antitubercular drugs, and the polio vaccine enabled the prevention and control of the many fatal infectious and parasitic diseases of previous eras. Throughout the 1950s and 1960s, a host of new medical techniques, technologies based on impressive complex machines, and organizational arrangements were introduced—for instance, heart pacemakers, kidney dialysis, open-heart surgery, and machine-dense intensive care units. Each new discovery was accompanied by excitement and the renewal of the hope of the conquest of disease by medical science. These new techniques and technologies have enabled the saving and extending of many lives, but the great promise envisioned in the 1940s and 1950s later became less optimistic. The anticipated successes of the earlier decade became fewer, and the unintended and unanticipated consequences of the medical technology became more apparent. Currently there are two highly publicized and interrelated concerns: the high cost of the medical technology and the increased hazards associated with the technology.

Among the general public, the growing concern with technology-associated medical hazards is due in part to a combination of consumer and ecology movements, furthered by media reports of sensational technology-related fatalities or harm. Indeed, practically every day the media report a new danger associated with a drug, a procedure, or a type of equipment (not to mention health dangers from environmental pollution produced by contemporary technology of one kind or another). Technology and the attendant damage it can do or does to humans are very much at the forefront of policy debates, including the heated debates about health policy (Wiener, Fagerhaugh, Strauss, and Suczek, 1980, 1982). The same arguments, of course, are going on within the hospitals. Great resources of personnel, skill, and organization are required to manage medical hazards. Establishing and maintaining an effective safety technology is rendered most difficult, given the myriad dangers produced in the hospital and their linkages to the related issues of cost containment and such moral and ethical issues as equity. This complexity of issues, as we shall see, poses perplexing choices not only for patients and their families but also for the health workers themselves.

Major Changes that Affect Health Care and Safety

We turn next to a consideration of major social and medical changes that together form the context within which clinical hazards arise and clinical safety work is done. There are at least two sets of these changes that affect safety work: (1) the character of contemporary illnesses (changing from acute to chronic illness) and (2) the impact of technology on health organizations and health practices.

Prevalence of Chronic Illness. The proliferation of medical technology is directly associated with the changing character of contemporary illness. Since the 1940s, industrially developed nations everywhere have manifested the same pattern of illness. Infectious and parasitic diseases have been largely controlled, and there have been increases in such chronic illnesses as cancer and cardiovascular, respiratory, renal, and endocrine diseases. Contemporary medical responses for chronic illnesses rely heavily on technology that is often applied simultaneously or in tandem to contain these diseases.

With regard to this technology, Lewis Thomas, an eminent cancer research physician, has popularized the term *halfway technology* (Thomas, 1974). By this he means medical interventions applied after the fact, either to make up for the incapacitating effects of a disease whose course one is unable to do much about or to postpone death. An outstanding example of this is the transplanting of organs. Thomas argues that this level of technology is by its nature highly sophisticated and at the same time primitive. The enormous technology involved in caring for heart disease, for example, includes specialized ambulances, diagnostic services, and patient care units with all kinds of electronic gadgets and an array of new, skilled health professionals to maintain the machines and the patients hooked to the machines. This type of technology is characteristically costly, calls for a continuing expansion of health facilities, and requires more and more highly trained personnel. Halfway technology continues until there is genuine understanding of the mechanism involved in disease, which as Thomas sees it means there should be more basic research to answer questions about mechanisms of disease in the various chronic illnesses. Until these questions are answered, he argues—correctly, in our view—that we must put up with halfway technology.

The fact that these illnesses cannot be "cured" but must be "managed" makes them different in many respects from acute illnesses around which health care was traditionally organized. By way of introduction to this difference, here is a brief look at the important qualities of chronic illness (Gerson and Strauss, 1975; Strauss, Fagerhaugh, Suczek, and Wiener, 1985). How they impact on patients' lives, on the work of health professionals, and on health institutions will be more apparent from the later discussion.

First, of course, chronic illnesses are long-term. Their long-term character requires repeated interactions over many months and years between patients and health workers. Second, chronic illnesses are uncertain in many ways. Often the prognosis is uncertain. The uncertainty can stem not only from the disease itself but also from the various medical interventions. This poses problems for long-range planning, not only for the professionals in disease management but for patients' long-range management of their lives. Third, and related to the uncertainty, many chronic illnesses are inherently episodic in nature: acute flare-ups followed by remission are not uncommon. This episodic nature restricts patients from leading "normal" lives and adds to the inability to effectively plan long-range. Fourth, chronic diseases require proportionally large efforts of palliation, relieving symptoms (such pain and discomforts as nausea and dizziness) and decreasing the disruption to normal bodily functioning (ambulating, eating, sleeping, eliminating, and so on). These palliative requirements are often multiple, because they may accompany the disease and/or the various medical and nursing measures to control the disease. The palliative efforts involve not only the professional staff but patients and their families as well. Not infrequently the effort required of family members may wreak havoc in a patient's household. Fifth, chronic illnesses are often multiple: many chronic diseases are systemic and degenerative; long-term breakdowns of one organ or system can affect other systems, and the uses of therapies to control one disease may produce other diseases (iatrogenic diseases). Sixth, chronic diseases are disproportionally intrusive upon the lives of patients. Patients' life-styles may be drastically altered by the illness itself, and/or the efforts required to control the diseases and to relieve symptoms often result in high social and financial costs to the families. Seventh, chronic diseases require a wide variety of ancillary services. Depending upon the illness and the complexity of the illness, large numbers of ancillary professionals are required, such as social and occupational workers, counselors, and people from other technical services. Eighth, chronic illnesses are expensive. Considering all the above characteristics even in the absence of elaborate and expensive technologies, the need for routine monitoring of the illness course, the occurrence of crises, and the need for ancillary services drives up the cost of care (Schroeder, Showstack, and Robert, 1979). Repeated hospitalizations and the complex character of chronic illness care imply proportionally greater outlay and administration costs for health organizations and funding agencies alike. Lastly, chronic diseases imply conflicts of authority among patients, health care and other service workers, and health care institutions themselves. Conflicts are not uncommon because there is inherent conflict of interest: physicians and nurses seek to control the character and quality of their work, patients seek to control their bodies and what happens to them, and health care services seek to control the flow of funds.

It is clear that halfway technologies have prolonged life but have also made patients and health professionals dependent on the technologies throughout the long years of a moderate to severe chronic illness. Patients enter a cycle that takes them through the hospital, back home, then to the clinic or physicians, back to the hospital in acute episode, and back again home. Problems of articulating the care given in the hospital, clinic, and home are immense. The technological explosion affects both the organizational structure of health care and the work of health professionals. In turn, the latter—the medical-nursing-technical work—affects the kind and quality of patient care.

Expansion of Medical Technology and Its Impact on Hospital Organization. Medical specialization and technological innovations have a special feature: they are parallel and interactive. Medical specialization leads to technological innovation; then, as a given technology is used, physicians and industrial designers collaborate to improve it. As it is refined, that process leads to ever more specialization and associated work and procedures.

The growth of intensive care units (ICUs) illustrates this progression. The first ICUs to develop were created to care for a variety of very acutely ill patients, including those with cardiac disease. Then, because cardiac disease is a major killer, large research funds were made available for further refinement of cardiovascular monitors, drug therapies, and diagnostic procedures, while separate cardiac care units were evolving. Simultaneously, units that specialized in diagnostic cardiac services, such as cardiac catheterization and cardiopulmonary function testing, were developed for adults and children. Corresponding to these developments, specialists in heart surgery developed sophisticated cardiac technology. In large medical centers, each medical specialty is beginning to have its own intensive care units: neurological ICU, respiratory ICU, and so on.

A second illustration is provided by the latest specialties to be influenced by advanced technology: obstetrics and especially pediatrics. Fetal monitoring machines were developed to pick up early signs of fetal distress in high-risk laboring mothers. Simultaneously, intensive care nurseries were developed as adult critical care machinery was refined and scaled down in size in order to care for the increased numbers of high-risk infants saved. Pediatrics then began to be differentiated into perinatology and neonatology, and these specialties spawned a cadre of medical subspecialties, such as pediatric cardiology and pediatric neurology.

The expansion of specialized departments and services in hospitals generates (1) the expansion of physical facilities, (2) the reallocation of workers and the integration of new skilled personnel into a continuously changing division of labor, and (3) the establishment of complex relationships among a multiplicity of hospital services and departments.

The rapid introduction of technologies and the associated growth of specialized services have resulted in obsolescence of the hospital's physical plant, space usage, machinery, health professional skills, and, indeed, virtually all institutional arrangements. Thus, expansion of physical facilities also leads in most acute care hospitals to an ever growing space crunch, each specialty fighting to hang on to its space and, if possible, to expand its space. The addition of new technology requires the reallocation of space and extensive remodeling. Hospital architecture becomes quickly archaic. Even with new types of hospital construction, architects face problems of building to meet future technology and to satisfy the multitude of specialized services with their requirements. Since new technologies are constantly produced and introduced, as one well-informed architect told us, the hospital spaces become obsolete within seven to ten years.

As new specialized services are added, new kinds of work and specialized new workers are required, calling for a continuously and often swiftly changing division of labor. The new work may involve reallocation of workers already employed and training them in new skills, or the integration of new workers whose work tends to overlap, or the integration of new workers whose work is totally unfamiliar to the existing workers. Interactional problems often result, as the new workers try to carve out roles and tasks that impinge on those of the workers employed longer. Generally, it takes some time to delineate the total picture so that each specialist can work efficiently with the others.

Changes in a respiratory therapy department at one hospital illustrate this point, in a pattern of change not uncommon elsewhere. In the late 1960s when respiratory machines became more complex and varied, and as their usage increased throughout the hospital, a special respiratory therapy department was established. Previously, nurses on one of the pediatric wards were trained to administer treatments, using these machines. Servicing of the equipment was then supervised by the central supply service of the nursing administration department. Those who worked with the machines were strictly "machine tenders." When the new special service was established, a certified respiratory therapist (RT) had to be hired. Some workers who were familiar with the equipment were retrained, becoming certified technicians under a grandfather clause. Responsibility for supervising the department was shifted to the anesthesia service of the medical department; later it shifted to the medical respiratory service. As the number of certified therapists increased, the department gradually took over respiratory treatments throughout the hospital. Old-timers in the department recalled their numerous misunderstandings with nurses and doctors. Some nurses had viewed them only as machine tenders. In turn, the RTs thought them neither properly trained to use the machines nor utilizing their expertise properly. Some nurses resented the RTs and preferred doing the treatment themselves, especially since the nurses could not control the timing of the treatments to fit their overall patient-care schedule. Optimum treatment outcomes require technician-nurse communication, so there was mutual accusation of each other for not sharing information about patients that was pertinent to care. In addition, the ordering of drugs used in conjunction with the machines is usually done by nurses. Often they did not realize this was their responsibility, and treatment was delayed. Physicians were confused about the RTs' capabilities. Sometimes a physician's therapeutic order was judged as inappropriate for the patient, so that physician-RT interactional difficulties were encountered in remedying the physician's order. Later, when the intensive care units expanded, RTs who were experienced in intensive care therapy were hired, as well as the existing workers were retrained.

Today in the hospital the confusion in tasks and roles of RTs on the health team has markedly decreased. Their specialized expertise is recognized, so much so that they now teach medical students and interns about the intricacies of operating the respiratory equipment. The last new addition to their department was that of an RT who was experienced in neonatal intensive care. This new specialist expressed anxiety about becoming accepted by the nursing staff, which was unfamiliar with her special skills. Since the infants were so fragile—with a small margin of error being possible—she feared she would have to prove herself a competent specialist to the nursing staff. We can see this same process of organizational change reflected in numerous articles related to the experiences of clinical nurse specialists, as they attempt to clarify their roles in the face of gaining the acceptance of nurses and other health professionals (Ayers, 1979; Piazza and Jackson, 1978; Woodrow and Bell, 1971; and Wyers, Grove, and Pastorino, 1985).

Rapid technological innovation also requires that the division of labor be constantly negotiated and renegotiated, as new technology is added or substituted for the old. Thus, when ICUs were first developed, they were staffed mainly by physicians and nurses. As the numbers of machines increased, not only in the unit itself but also in related services, and as the larger numbers and varied kinds of critical care patients increased, then either new tasks were assigned to the existing skilled personnel or new skilled personnel were required. Now respiratory therapists are part of the ICU team, and an army of new and already employed skilled personnel stream into the unit providing essential services, like those of the electronic technician, bioengineer, laboratory technician, x-ray technician, and safety engineer. This incorporation of new categories of skilled workers is taking place simultaneously all over the hospital and in many ancillary service departments.

Accompanying the rapid technological incorporation has been a parallel expansion of ancillary services. The explosion of numbers, kinds, and models of machinery on the wards makes the purchase of equipment and supplies a more complex process. It requires consultation from a variety of sources because of the specialized technology and its accompanying safety issues. Also, the processes of procuring, storing, and distributing supplies, equipment, and equipment parts throughout the hospital are increasing in magnitude and complexity. Indeed, the traffic of patients, workers, equipment, and carts in most large acute care hospitals is striking—witness the frequent traffic jams at the elevators. The increased volume of goods, equipment, and supplies has brought in still another category of worker: the material management and transport engineer (Housley, 1978). A concern for environmental safety has brought into existence the environmental safety departments: these are responsible for interpreting safety codes to the hospital administration and to the total hospital services, especially high-technology services, and for monitoring patient and worker safety. In large institutions, the safety department is becoming differentiated into finer specialty units (electro-safety, biochemical safety, radiation safety), in response to the explosion of drug and equipment technology and the many safety regulations pertaining to their use.

As a consequence of diagnostic and treatment services becoming increasingly differentiated into finer and finer specialties, there are further problems of articulating work within each department and service, as well as of articulating the various services (Georgopoulos and Mann, 1978). So one often finds a bewildering profusion of task forces, standing committees, and informal meetings, both intra- and interdepartmental, that are attempts to coordinate the work. Not unexpectedly, a recent trend seems to point to an increase in middle management and liaison nurses, whose main responsibilities include both the coordinating of intradepartmental/interdepartmental work and the troubleshooting of actual deficiencies in organizational coordination.

Given all this, the hospital administrators face the awesome tasks of coordinating a multitude of specialty departments and services, as well as coping with multitudes of regulations and regulatory agencies in order to stay in operation (Somer, 1969), arbitrating demands by competing specialized services for equipment and resources, and at the same time attempting to contain costs. To attain some measure of order and efficiency, administrators have turned to data computerization. But again, this technology requires specialized skilled workers. Parallel to all of this is a search for organizational and administrative theories to bring order to the chaos. A variety of theories abound, among them the general systems theory (Kast and Rosenzweig, 1966), matrix theory (Neuhauser, 1972), contingency theory (Mockler, 1971), and participative decision-making theory (Lowin, 1968). They are all theoretically interesting but do not always seem to provide pragmatic answers. Understandably, then, the rapidly changing conditions created by new technologies, new regulations, and new community pressure groups mean that "management by ad hoc-ing" or "by putting out fires" becomes the frequent administrative mode of operation.

This development of technological specialization within hospitals has had a ripple effect on related health care services, such as the clinics and home care agencies. The high cost of hospital care has meant that more and more services must be offered through ambulatory clinics, which have had to specialize to meet these needs. In the clinics, as the hospitals, new personnel must be integrated, with all the attendant problems of working out a division of labor and forging a team to get the job done. With increasing numbers of chronically ill patients being sustained at home by means of such medical technology as pulmonary and dialysis machines, special treatment procedures, and drugs, home care agencies are also having to meet the demands for specialized services and are employing pulmonary, cardiovascular, and cancer nursing specialists. Furthermore, work from the hospital, the clinic, and the home health services must be coordinated. This has created still other categories of nurses: the patient discharge coordinator, the cancer or respiratory liaison nurse, and so on.

The fact that life can now be sustained and prolonged to a degree not possible two decades ago poses great problems for workers in these services. These dilemmas have necessitated still another category of specialist, the bioethicist, in large medical centers. The ethical dilemmas, together with the intensity of work and the frustration of coping with complex bureaucratic organizations, have created a technologically related work hazard: "burnout" (Freudenberger, 1974; Maslach, 1976; Shubin, 1978). To cope with the hazards of burnout and stress, staff are also consulting specialists who utilize "soft technology," as represented by the work of psychiatrists, psychiatric nurse specialists, and psychiatric social workers.

Although most of the above discussion pertains to large medical centers, the rate of technological migration to smaller hospitals and communities is also becoming increasingly rapid (Russell, 1979). This diffusion to smaller hospitals is due to several factors: the increased role of industry in medical technology and its need to expand the market, the supply of trained personnel from large research and training centers who are seeking opportunities to practice their skills, the prestige requirement and the competition of hospitals for attracting patients and physicians, and the demand that services and resources be distributed equitably among all citizens. In smaller hospitals, the impact of technology on hospital structure and work—and on safety/hazard—differs only in rate and intensity.

Technology's Impact on Chronic Illness Care. The acceleration of specialization with its subsequent creation of complex bureaucratic health structures has resulted in (1) a fragmentation of chronic care that involves more possibilities of discontinuity of care and the accompanying accusations of "dehumanization"; (2) a further incorporation of new workers and roles to remedy the ill effects of fragmented care and dehumanization; (3) new social and psychological problems for health workers, patients, and their families; (4) the generation of a need for "soft technology"—the expertise of psychiatrists and psychiatric nurse specialists—for managing the social and psychological problems; and (5) a reaction against technology in the form of new care modalities.

The fragmentation effects of specialization arise because multitudes of departments and layers and layers of workers must be coordinated within the chain of tasks necessary to complete a treatment or a diagnostic test. When carrying out the tasks, the patient may be neglected, because each department has its own specific situation in which work can go awry. Because much has been written about the fragmentation of health care and the depersonalizing effects on patients (Howard, 1975), health professionals are becoming sensitive to these untoward effects and are trying to remedy them by adding liaison workers and fashioning new roles, such as those of the primary nurse (Mundinger, 1973), primary physician (Andreopoulos, 1974), and patient advocate (Hamil, 1976). These efforts are commendable and must be continued, but given the organizational considerations outlined earlier, remedying the overall situation is extremely difficult. An added complication is that the intricate technologies require very specialized knowledge from many experts who may not agree at all with one another. Moreover, the effects of various medical interventions are uncertain, and there is concern about the possibility of iatrogenic disease.

Meanwhile, at home the chronically ill and their families bear the major responsibility for management during the non-acute phases of illness. This may require teaching them the intricacies of operating a machine and giving them advice on dietary restrictions, medications to take, possible side effects to watch for, and life-style changes that patient and family may have to make. New community resources and new forms of patient-professional interactions must be created to assist the patient in managing the medical regimen and in living with a disability.

Among the social and psychological problems for the ill people and their families are the stresses of living with the constant threat of death, carrying on in the midst of seemingly never ending responsibilities to monitor and manage the complex regimen, or coping with social isolation and bodily disfigurement. In response to these problems there has been a proliferation of support, such as death counseling and many other types of groups. Clearly, the hard technology applied to control chronic diseases has generated a need for the seemingly discrepant soft technology: the group work and counseling skills of psychiatrists, psychiatric nurses, social workers, psychologists and so on, as well as of lay workers. Soft technology is necessary not only for professionals using hard technology, in order to help them maintain their composure and equanimity, but also for the receivers of the hard technology: the sick and their kin.

A reaction has set in against current medical institutions and their highly technologized practices, as evidenced by the growth of such alternative health care approaches as natural birth centers and holistic health centers. In general, these alternative approaches are peripheral to the traditional medical institutions but are beginning to be incorporated into them; for instance, alternative birth centers now exist side by side with traditional medical obstetrical departments in hospitals.

Technology as Affected by Political, Economic, and Social Concerns

A number of political, social, and economic concerns enter into any discussion of medical technology. Among the major ones are the high cost of medical technology, the safety of technologies, and the moral concerns. These are often inter-related issues, and they are subject to much debate by many groups (Wiener, Fagerhaugh, Strauss, and Suczek, 1982).

Of current concern and debate is the high cost of medical care, of which medical technology is often named as the major culprit (Altman and Blandon, 1979). Some blame this high cost on competition for profit, on physicians' avarice, and on hospitals' drive for prestige (Ehrenreich and Ehrenreich, 1971; Starr, 1982; Waitzkin and Waterman, 1974). Hence the hue and cry against the danger of the "medical-industrial complex" (Ehrenreich and Ehrenreich, 1971; Relman, 1980b). Others argue that competition will reduce costs. The search for the causes of high medical costs clearly relates to who should bear the burden of paying them, which in turn raises the moral question of equity. The demand for equity implies a fair distribution of medical resources, so that comprehensive health care—which includes prevention, diagnostic, therapeutic, and rehabilitative services—is provided for all citizens. The issue of just how comprehensive this care should be is, of course, hotly debated.

A second consideration is that the general public, health workers, governmental agencies, and the health industry are all involved with the medical technologies. Safety regulations applying to the hospitals run into the thousands. They cover the work of every area and department: the hospital's use of space, the building of new space, its electric outlets, oxygen installation, transporting of material and people, thousands of drugs and hundreds of pieces of equipment, disposal of chemical and nuclear waste, and so on. These requirements originate in many levels of government (federal, state, county, and city) and in many departments of the government (Ivancevich, 1977). Other regulations come from within the health industry, from various professional organizations governing the practice and conduct of their members, and from the American Hospital Association itself. These regulations are lobbied for and against, and fought over (often with every political means possible) by the various groups. Thus, debates rage about whether there is too much or too little regulation, and about what constitutes appropriate evidence of certification of need for hospitals that want a given innovation, reasonable limitations on a researcher's freedom, or tolerable risk. In industry, there are complaints that governmental safety regulations increase costs and that the bureaucratic system is contrary to the spirit of free enterprise. Among researchers, the regulations are felt to be a roadblock to scientific inquiry and medical breakthroughs (Roy, 1978). The counterposition is that industry is using this argument to cover up its profit motive and to avoid governmental interference. Moral rationales are applied by opposing groups to support their positions.

A third consideration pertains to the moral concerns associated with the argument that technology is at the root of what is perceived as the current dehumanization of medical care (Illich, 1977; Kennedy, 1976). There are bioethical discussions of such topics as informed consent, sustaining life at the expense of enormous social and economic strains for the family and society, the extent to which genetics should be tampered with, and the right to die (Mann, 1970; Davis and Aroskar, 1983; Jameton, 1984). Moral considerations also enter the debate on cost, leading to such questions as: Is the cost of technology worth the benefits to be gained from using it? Who is worthy to receive costly medical care? And perhaps most important of all, who shall decide?

In our pluralistic society, many individuals and groups within the general public, the health professions, and the health industry take positions on one or more of these concerns. These actors vary in terms of the stakes involved, their self-interests, and their ideologies. From those varying perspectives, social diagnoses are made, and the major culprits responsible for the chaotic state of our health care system are identified. Because the many special-interest groups hold widely divergent views about health problems, they find it extremely difficult to resolve either the debates or the profound problems inextricably linked with both medical technology and chronic illness. Meanwhile, medical knowledge and medical technology continue to advance and help to increase the numbers of chronically ill at home, in hospitals, in clinics, and nursing homes—and thus infinitely multiply the problems addressed.

Technological Assessment

The foregoing discussion emphasizes the complex risk/ benefit questions about medical technology that must be resolved. In short, what are the benefits to be derived from given technologies, but with which risks? (The risks are clinical, social, cost, legal, and moral, as they affect equity, patients, families, health professionals, institutions, and society in general.) The concern over risks and benefits spurred efforts to assess medical technology during the late 1960s, but not without many obstacles in doing so. The primary focus throughout the 1970s and 1980s has been on cost, the appropriate and effective use of technology, and whether some technologies, such as computed axial tomography (CAT) scans, ICUs, and organ transplants, actually justify their cost. Assessment of the social impact of technologies—their effects on patients' and families' ''quality of life,'' and on legal, moral-ethical, and dehumanization issues—has been a secondary focus.

The adequacy of assessing medical technology rests on a set of assumptions about its effectiveness and reliability. These are based on well-established criteria on which safety-danger benefits and effectiveness can be established, as well as on the assurance that methods and tools for evaluation are reliable. Equally important is the degree to which the various parties can achieve consensus, not only on assessment methodologies but also on their priorities and need. The parties concerned with technological assessment include research and development groups, industrial companies, health professionals, health care institutions, health insurance companies, health policymakers, patients, and other consumers of health care. All have different stakes in the debate and its outcome.

A number of governmental and nongovernmental groups are involved in various aspects of technological assessment. More than a dozen federal agencies conduct or support biomedical research. Various professional associations have also developed their own medical technological assessment groups (Office of Technology Assessment, 1978). New agencies concerned solely with technological assessment were created through legislative action. In 1972, the Office of Technology Assessment (OTA) was established to help legislative policymakers anticipate and plan for potential effects—whether beneficial or harmful—of technology applications. In 1978, the National Center for Health Care Technology was established to undertake studies to identify issues and consequences related to the development and application of effective, efficient, and safe technology.

Most of the technological assessment has been done by governmental and quasi-governmental organizations, such as the Office of Technology Assessment, the National Institutes of Health, and the National Academy of Sciences. Among physicians, the acceptance of assessment has been slow. In fact, the term *technology assessment* did not enter the lexicon of Index Medicus until 1978. Indeed, there was strong opposition to assessment from organized medicine and the manufacturers of equipment. This, together with the economic cuts imposed by the Reagan administration, resulted in the demise of the National Center for Health Care Technology (Jennett, 1986; Perry, 1982).

Aside from the problems of opposition by parties concerned with assessment, there is the obstacle of evaluating methodologies for assessing technologies (Jennett, 1986). A study by the Office of Technology Assessment (1976) took a pessimistic view of the state of technological assessment with regard to developing policies for effective and economic application of technologies. According to this study, the methodologies available to determine technological assessment are disappointing. The OTA reports list at least four basic methodological limitations:

- The field is new and therefore lacking in standard, usable methods, especially when quality of life and moral-ethical issues are involved.
- Medical technologies are very diverse and complicated, and thus standard formats for assessments are difficult to achieve.
- Technology assessments are hampered by weaknesses in the tools and techniques of social sciences that must be used to calculate social impacts.
- Groups carrying out assessment have had great difficulty establishing boundaries for their studies.

These deficiencies are being remedied as the need is becoming more apparent (Jennett, 1986).

A second obstacle is that technology assessment can be very costly and time-consuming (Coates, 1972; Relman, 1982). Cost is high because a large sample must be included, cooperation of geographically distant hospitals must be enlisted, special systems may have to be created to transport specimens, additional personnel need to be employed at the various hospitals to perform the necessary administrative or laboratory tasks, and the evaluation team must travel frequently over long distances (McDermott, 1977; Byars and others, 1978; Ederer, 1975). Clinical evaluation is a formidable cost issue not only for the users of technology but for the producers of technology as well.

A third obstacle to technology assessment is the vested interests of medical practice and medical research that hinder objective evaluation of medical technologies. Schroeder and Showstack (1977) have argued persuasively that the continued debates about the appropriate types of mastectomy to use for breast cancer and the controversy over cost-benefit of coronary care units and coronary artery bypass surgery exist primarily because users are reluctant to evaluate the technology, *their* technology, in question. This results in a paucity of good evaluation reports. Further, they add that the nature of research support, both public and private, is a further barrier to good evaluation. For example, America's single largest biomedical research agency, the National Institutes of Health (NIH), accounts for almost two-thirds of the federal expenditures for health research. The categorical nature of NIH with its eleven separate institutes and its representative disciplinary study section, plus the systematic incentive toward "protechnology," create a powerful disincentive to cross-disciplinary technology evaluation.

Moreover, institutions may experience unfavorable financial consequences should an evaluation be unfavorable. For example, the introduction of a new technology, such as the computerized tomography (CT) scanner, can produce a threefold increase in radiology billings. Thus there is an institutional reluctance to conclude that the technology is unnecessary for a favorable patient care outcome (Knaus, Schroeder, and Davis, 1977).

Relman (1980b), the editor of the *New England Journal of Medicine,* has criticized the free enterprise approach to technical problems. His criticism was directed against the "new medical-industrial complex," an aggregate of proprietary hospitals and medicine. He maintained that the combination of hospital and physicians in a business partnership tends to overemphasize those technological procedures that are profitable over those that are necessary or beneficial.

Related to the above considerations is a fourth obstacle to effective technological assessment. Socioeconomic "protechnology" factors tend to generate a greater use of technology without its appropriate evaluation. Schroeder (1979) cites the following protechnology factors that stimulated the use of tests and procedures during the 1960 and 1970s: (1) the physician reimbursement (fee-for-service) system that encouraged a large financial incentive favoring technology-intensive medical practice; (2) an increased physician specialization with associated specialized procedures and equipment, coupled with a surplus of physicians; (3) the tendency of new techniques and technology to be additive rather than substitutive (for example, x-ray and ultrasound); (4) a surplus of acute care hospital beds that stimulate hospitals to compete for physicians by acquiring new technology; (5) the cost-plus reimbursement system of most hospitals; (6) the extensive coverage of acute hospital care by third-party insurances; (7) the reluctance of physicians to abandon hope for incurable patients or cease treating them with medical technologies; (8) the reward system of medical academia that promotes technology evaluation as a scholarly activity; (9) the ease of capital formation for acquiring new technologies; and (10) the malpractice threat. (Factors 5, 6, and 9 are less relevant today due to the changes made in the financial reimbursement system by the DRGs and the regulatory measures instituted to control the diffusion of technology in medical practice.) All of these forces interact, thereby encouraging the extensive use of technology. Because of these factors, plus the great difficulties encountered in evaluating technology, a considerable number of technologies are established and used before their inadequacies are widely suspected. Consequently, while the necessarily lengthy process of evaluation is proceeding, new technologies continue to flood the marketplace.

All of this, coupled with a greater public interest in medical technological development, is fanned by the media and increases the desire for equity and access to medical technology. At the same time, the public is rarely told of problems involved in evaluating these new technologies, including their safety or the current clinical disfavor associated with particular technologies. Then there is also our legal system, which tends to reflect a populist view that technology is obviously good and that regulations should not limit the right to access to expensive procedures no matter how high the cost and how small the benefits (Freishtat, 1982).

By the 1980s, physicians and medical equipment producers decreased their resistance to technology assessment. This change has been attributed to hospitals' efforts at cost control and medical practice control during the 1970s (Jennett, 1986). Among those efforts have been the passage of the Professional Standard Review Organization and the establishment of the Utilization Review Commission in 1974. These efforts brought about data collection from hospital records, including records of diagnosis, therapeutic procedures, length of hospital stay, and so on, as well as review of the records by physicians, often members of the hospital staff. Such reviews assure that services paid for by Medicare and Medicaid have been delivered at appropriate institutions with reasonable standards of care. Such audits have made public the variations among doctors' practices and the need for a more uniform standard of practice. These efforts have been augmented by standards imposed by the Joint Commission on Accreditation of Hospitals.

In 1981, through the enactment of the Diagnostic Related Group (DRGs) by the federal government, hospital reimbursement on a retrospective basis was eliminated. Under the new system, hospitals were reimbursed by a prospective policy that set limits on technology usage and on days of hospitalization, for 467 related groups of diseases. Hospitals and physicians not using the technology appropriately and economically were penalized. These stringent financial controls compelled physicians and hospitals to reexamine standards of practice and usage of technology. Consequently, there were pleas for governmental evaluation of technology (Iglehart, 1983), as well as a call for federal funds and the establishment of a commission to evaluate technology (Bunker, Fowles, and Schaffarzich, 1981; Relman, 1980a, 1982). Ironically, the American Medical Association (AMA) and the Health Industry Manufacturers Association, each of which had contributed to the demise of the National Center for Health Care Technology, were both asking for legislation to assess technology. The AMA in 1983 established its own mechanism to assess technology (Jones, 1983).

Gradually there has grown an acceptance for the need of mechanisms to establish consensus on the use of technologies. There is now general agreement that at a minimum there should be a mechanism for an information clearinghouse (Committee for Evaluating Medical Technology in Clinical Practice, 1985). Efforts at reaching consensus among practitioners on the appropriate application of technology for various illness conditions have gradually increased also.

In sum, technology assessment is highly political, even though there has been a gradually growing consensus as to its need. The many social, economic, and political factors exert pressures for development and use of medical technologies before their appropriateness and efficiency are determined, even before the grounds for their increased use are established. Combining those pressures with the many difficulties in assessing the safety of technologies, the safe use of technology becomes additionally problematic. When inadequately assessed, the technologies pose difficulties for predicting either long-term or unfavorable risks. Hence, many ambiguities and unknowns accompany the use of equipment and procedures. This situation places a heavy burden on health professionals in their attempts at maximizing clinical safety.

Dominance of Safety Work and Consequent Dilemmas

Hospitals are potentially dangerous places. First of all, patients are already in an endangered illness state when they first enter the hospital. In order to control or reverse the illness, many machines, equipment, and drugs may be simultaneously and sequentially utilized. All are of potential risk to the patient. Workers can also endanger the patient through lack of proper skills, errors, or for very human reasons, such as being tired. The technologized physical environment can endanger both the patient and worker: for instance, there is a potential for electrical shock and burns, due to incorrectly connected or malfunctioning machinery, explosion of inflammable gases, or leakages of noxious chemical gases. Crowded space and high noise level can lead to errors.

A tremendous organization of support services is required to assure hazard minimization. This includes machine repair and maintenance, supply lines for goods and services, and orientation and in-service programs to upgrade workers' skills. Also, the increased specialization of services requires that layers and layers of workers be coordinated in the chain of tasks needed to complete a treatment or a diagnostic procedure. There is always a possibility for delay or error all along the chain of tasks. Thus, institutional misarrangements or nonarrangements of essential services can lead to hazards. All of these potential sources are linked, so a malfunctioning in one can potentially affect others. These linkages will become more apparent in the next chapters.

Indeed, it is safe to say that hospitals are basically organized around danger-risk-safety considerations. Acute care hospitals are grouped as primary, secondary, and tertiary hospitals. Tertiary hospitals are those that treat patients in highly dangerous illness states, where a number of experimental technologies are utilized. In different workplaces within the hospital, potential sources of hazards and their dimensions are taken into account when allocating resources. Aside from special medical and surgical units, hospital care units are broken down into critical care units, intermediate units, and rehabilitation or extended care units. Obviously, critical care units command the greatest resources in the hospital, because of their many sources of dangers and risks, and because their probability for hazards is potentially high.

We should add that hazards are not only physical but can endanger the interactions among staff members and with patients. Also they can endanger the identities of all persons involved. Highly technologized hospitals with all of their potential sources of hazards also increase the stresses on health workers. Stresses are produced by the rapid work pace, the frustrations of coping with a highly complex and bureaucratic work situation, and the difficulties of balancing moral-ethical issues, such as keeping someone alive while prolonging suffering. So the identities of personnel may further suffer. In addition, all of these consequences may affect staff morale and "sentimental order"— the intangible but very real patterning of mood and sentiment that characteristically exists on each ward (Glaser and Strauss, 1965). This effect in turn can lower the quality of patient care and increase the clinical hazards of giving that care.

Yet the improvement in therapeutic technology, even though "halfway," now enables the stretching out of the lives of the chronically ill. The stretching occurs not only at the aging end but at the birthing end as well. Many premature and congenitally defective infants are saved, and this adds to the pool of chronically ill people. The stretching out results in much uncertainty about the management of dangers and risks. As lives are extended, multiple body systems may deteriorate, thus calling for multiple kinds of therapeutic and palliative measures that carry potential risks. Moreover, hazard management is complicated further because efforts to control one hazard may have deleterious effects on another—or even create a new disease.

Safety Arenas and the Balancing of Hazards

The net effect of rapid technological expansion has enlarged the hospital arena, through both the segmentation of traditional health professionals and the addition of new groups of health and lay workers who may share or disagree about any aspect of health care, including its dangers and risks. Groups concerned with cost, safety regulations, equity, and bioethical issues are intruding more and more into the hospital arena, which is no longer an island unto itself. As noted in our discussion of the

political, economic, and social forces impinging on the health
care system, other arenas affect the hospital: the health care industry (drugs and instrumentations), the various social movements (patient self-care, women, holistic), the institutions (federal, state, and county regulatory agencies), and the professional
movements (organizational and intellectual). Thus they affect
the structure and the work of health care personnel.

Issues involving safety management can also be viewed
as constituting a safety arena. Given the many kinds and types
of potential hazards and the growing complexity of hospital
organization, the management of hazards provokes constant
discussion, debate, and negotiation among representatives of
the various interested parties. (*Negotiation* here means the constant process of bargaining, working out disagreements, and
creating alliances among the various implicated groups; see
Strauss, 1978, 1982. This negotiative aspect will be discussed
more fully in our last chapter.) Although all hospital personnel
are concerned with some aspect of safety, any consensus as to
which hazards are of priority—and the how, when, and the who
of assuring the safety—is often difficult to reach. This is due
to the increased differentiation of workers, with each group of
workers developing and possessing different competencies, identities, language, values, and interests (Bucher and Strauss, 1961;
Hughes, 1971).

Debates and dissensions are apt to arise because each
group will be balancing different dangers and what it is willing
to risk. For example, hospital administrators tend to weigh cost
against danger prevention, while physicians are less concerned
with cost but are mostly concerned with weighing and balancing various medical dangers. Nurses are concerned additionally
with patients' psychosocial risks and the sentimental order of
wards.

The balancing also involves weighing the consequences
of various actions and what may be risked by them. The risks
may engender legal repercussions, with a negative impact on
individual careers and hospital reputations. In our highly litigious society, hospital workers are now concerned with being
sued for negligence. Not uncommonly, doctors complain of hav-

ing to practice "defensive medicine" to protect themselves against potential suits. Yet, defensive practice often exposes patients to unnecessary and costly diagnostic and treatment procedures.

The interrelatedness of the various institutional and career risks can be illustrated by the following example. A prominent pediatric cardiac surgeon was recruited to a large medical center because his presence would add to its reputation. Part of the bargain in recruiting him was a promise that the hospital would not only obtain new technology but also give him an office space in the nursing ward. Hospital space was remodeled to accommodate the new technology and to provide office space and a storage room for his equipment. His surgical technology involved doing pioneer surgery on high-risk children. He and his assisting physicians were concerned with working out the complex medical risks associated with the new technology. Since the technology was very new, the resulting fatalities were rather high. Nurses lost their composure because of the pressures due to learning new skills for coping with the medical hazards. They also had to deal with their anxieties regarding the many deaths. Their morale plunged, and they began to question the bioethics of the new technology. Moreover, during a routine safety check, the fire marshal noted that the hallways were cluttered with equipment because the storage room was no longer available. He became alarmed, for putting all the equipment in the hallway entailed a breaking of safety regulations. If there were a fire, removing the patients would be difficult.

This graphic example illustrates not only the different risks and dangers being balanced by various groups of workers but also the degree to which each group could be relatively unaware of the safety concerns of the others. The example also illustrates the host of organizational arrangements that may be required to minimize hazards.

Summary

There is a basic dilemma in the ensuring of clinical safety within hospitals. Despite the staff's intensive focus on safety and an emphasis on the "errorless imperative," there are many factors that militate against assurance of complete safety. Among these factors are the nature of the chronic illnesses themselves, the characteristics of contemporary medical technology, the impact of both on hospital organization, the variety of perspectives and skills of the personnel, and the discrepant views on some basic issues pertaining to clinical safety and the work of maximizing it.

2

⌁⌁⌁⌁⌁⌁⌁⌁⌁⌁⌁⌁⌁⌁⌁⌁⌁⌁⌁⌁⌁⌁⌁⌁⌁⌁

The Trajectory of Illness:
A Framework for Organizing
and Managing Clinical Safety

Since hospitalized patients are frequently in very unstable acute phases of their diseases that are managed with potentially risky treatments, a central concern of the personnel is to minimize and control the clinical risks. To understand how they do this, we have developed the concept of trajectory safety. This emphasizes the organizational, interactional, and work aspects of the staff's efforts—as well as those of the patients.

Illness Trajectory

We turn first in this chapter to a central analytic distinction between two terms, a *course of illness* and what we shall call an *illness trajectory* (Glaser and Strauss, 1968; Fagerhaugh and Strauss, 1977; Strauss and others, 1984; Strauss, Fagerhaugh, Suczek, and Wiener, 1985). Illness *course* is the health professional's term that refers to the diagnosing and treating of illness. The term implies that each kind of illness has its specific pathologies, that there are more or less characteristic phases with matching symptoms, and that medical and nursing interventions will reverse, halt, or slow down the disease process. In contrast, *trajectory* refers not only to the physiological unfolding of the patient's illness but to the total organization of work done over that illness course, as well as the impact on those involved with that work and its organization, which in turn affects their work and, not incidentally, the illness course itself. For different illnesses, the associated trajectories involve different medical and nursing actions, different kinds of skills and other resources, and a different parcelling out of tasks among the workers (including perhaps kin and patient). Trajectories also involve quite different relationships—instrumental and expressive—among workers.

The term *trajectory* may at first be construed as just another label, a redundancy, if it is believed that existing conceptual formulations currently guiding professional practice can adequately incorporate elements conceptualized by trajectory. It can be further argued that such terms as *psychosocial aspects* or *psychosocial component* of patient care take into account more than the purely medical aspect of care. Yet, despite an implicit subsuming of the psychosocial component of patient care within the term *course of illness*, the medical perspective still dominates the views and activities of patient care. At acute care hospitals this is especially true, because of the acuity of illnesses and the consequent dominance of physicians in these settings. The organization-work-interactional focus of the term *trajectory* takes into account that health care occurs within an organized work setting. There many kinds and levels of workers, with their different interests, are involved in carrying out sequences of expected tasks in efforts to control illness.

Health professionals tend not to see their own actions, or that of the patients, as work. Rather, professionals' actions are seen as "interventions." Patients are seen as "clients" or "consumers" to whom services are rendered or whose "needs" are met. Terms such as *client* and *consumers* tend to connote passive recipients who do not actively work in their own behalf (Chang, 1980; Conway-Rutowsky, 1982)—not as sentient, ill persons who do just that. Along with some health professionals, various social scientists (Jobling, 1976; Johnson, 1977; Stacey, 1976) have criticized this view of patients as passive recipients of care and call for more patient control over patient care. However, they do not analyze the work of patients in quite the same way as we have, and not in the context of chronic illness (Strauss, Fagerhaugh, Suczek, and Wiener, 1982, 1985).

The concept of trajectory systematically takes into account conflicting perspectives among health team members in an effort to understand how patient care is organized, as well as the numerous contingencies affecting the organization of that care. The concept helps in the analytic ordering of the many varieties of events that occur when staff, patients, and kin attempt to control and cope with illness.

To do this and cope with illness, there must be an organization of work that involves a sequence of expected tasks. These are sometimes routinized, but even so they are subject to unexpected contingencies. These can arise from the illness itself as well as the diagnostic and therapeutic procedures. They also originate from organizational sources, and from biographical and life-style sources associated with the patient, family, and health care personnel themselves (Wiener, Fagerhaugh, Strauss, and Suczek, 1979). Unexpected contingencies are often difficult to control, but when combined with the nature of illness work, which involves work with people, the management of an illness trajectory is rendered highly complex and often highly problematic. As noted earlier, illness care requires working on and through the patient; hence a patient's reaction can affect the work. Also, patients participate in the work; that is, they are also workers, even in the hospital setting.

Routine and Problematic Trajectories

In any acute care hospital the patient population is experiencing varying types of trajectories. Some trajectories are relatively routine, such as those associated with appendectomy or hernia repair; the courses of illness and their phases are relatively specific, predictable, unambiguous, and of short duration. With other trajectories, the course and phases may be highly unpredictable, problematic, and of long duration. In addition, the patients are in varying phases of their extended chronic trajectories: at the beginning or middle, or in final phases.

In order to efficiently manage these varied trajectories, which involve both the illness and the work, hospitals generally are organized around professionals' work expectations with regard to similar types or phases of trajectories. For example, some wards are organized around similar types of trajectories according to medical specialties and subspecialties, while other wards are organized around phases of illness—such as the intensive care, intermediate and self-care units, and the surgical-recovery units for the immediate postoperative phase of surgical trajectories. Quite often, units are organized around work requirements that are associated with the degree of danger stemming from the types of illnesses themselves.

For the routine trajectories, the physicians, nurses, and other health personnel have a general knowledge of what will be the overall shape of the trajectory and what are the potential hazards involved in each phase. Hospital wards are equipped to handle these anticipated hazards with efficiency, using standard operating procedures. The coordination of resources and services for carrying out the necessary work to keep the trajectory on course is relatively easy. Of course, even with routine trajectories, unexpected contingencies can bring about an altered course. Such contingencies include unexpected drug reactions or patients refusing to participate in necessary medical or nursing procedures. However, with routine trajectories certain contingencies are to be anticipated, so that when they occur, they can be handled easily.

As previously mentioned, during the last several decades the numbers of patients with problematic trajectories have been increasing dramatically at acute care hospitals. Furthermore, the explosions of medical knowledge and technologies have produced a ''trajectory stretch-out,'' both at the beginning and aging periods of life. To illustrate the latter point: children with cystic fibrosis who would have died at early ages a decade ago now live longer because of the assistance of very complex medical regimens, though the disease is inevitably fatal. Of course, the stretch-out has been most notable at the aging end. Thus, acute care hospitals have high numbers of patients who are sixty-five years or older. In terms of acuity of illness then, hospitalized patients are often in serious illness states during the later phases of the extended trajectories. Then the numbers of improved technologies enable the patients to survive, so it has been predicted that by the 1990s acute care hospitals will turn into huge intensive care units (Levine, E., 1980). Given the recent trends toward building an expanded network of clinics, ambulatory surgical centers, emergency centers, and so on, this is very likely to be so.

In addition to the increased acuity of illness in hospitals, the trajectory stretch-out has resulted in diseases involving multiple body systems associated with the progression of diseases or with aging. Thus, a not uncommon type of patient is someone admitted to the hospital with ulcers and infected toes, due to a complication and a progression of diabetes that in turn involves the cardiovascular and renal systems, along with visual impairment, decreased mental acuity, and degenerative arthritis. Stabilizing such a patient's multiple illnesses or reversing or slowing down a potentially dangerous illness state are often highly problematic possibilities, because of the many kinds of unexpected contingencies associated with both the illness and the treatments. The various procedures, drugs, and machinery used to control illnesses may produce unexpected, untoward effects. Medical and nursing interventions done to control one disease may be incompatible or may negatively affect another illness. Thus, these contingencies pose difficulties in keeping multiple illnesses on course and in predicting their future phases. Also, the multiplicity of illnesses along with the many technologies required to keep them on course necessitates increased numbers of specialized personnel, as well as the complex organized resources upon which they draw. Organizational contingencies that create the miscoordination or lack of coordination of resources can also negatively affect the evolving trajectory.

Another characteristic of new technologies when used to control a trajectory is their many uncertainties and associated problems. Considerable experience and time are required to "work out the bugs" when perfecting a procedure, using a drug, operating a machine, or understanding how the various technologies interact and impact on body systems. The organization of the associated work takes time and experience, too. The history of new surgical procedures and new equipment, such as heart pacemakers and renal dialysis machines, gives ample

evidence of the relatively long period usually required for dealing with attendant uncertainties and problems. Moreover, this
affects trajectory management at home as well, for the chronic
illnesses are often characterized by both acute and nonacute
periods that necessitate the ill and their families be responsible
for management at home during the usually lengthier nonacute
phases. A regimen may require learning about the proper administration of drugs and their side effects, the various procedures for using machinery, as well as the indicators designating
when the trajectory is out of control and when professional help
should be sought.

The very rapidity of technological innovation has generated a continuous flow of new kinds of problematic trajectories.
As soon as the technology catches up with such a trajectory,
the next round of technology is likely to have the same destabiliz-
ing effect. In large medical centers, where much of the new
technology is developed, this process is never ending. For professionals, there is the exhilaration felt at mapping out the illness phases and controlling the challenging illness courses. Yet
it exists side by side with the many stresses engendered by coping with uncertainty and all the problems associated with problematic trajectories.

Generally speaking, trajectory management is often fraught
with such problems, given the many contingencies stemming
from the illnesses themselves, from the various medical interventions, and from organizational and other external sources—
some anticipated, but only a portion relatively controllable. Indeed, the word *management* neither adequately describes the full
complexity of trajectory work nor the consequences for all who
work at controlling the trajectory. More appropriate terms for
the handling of such problematic trajectories are that they are
"shaped" and "experienced" (Strauss, Fagerhaugh, Suczek,
and Wiener, 1985). *Shaping* refers to the fact that staffs handle
the contingencies as best they can, although they are far from
having full control of the trajectory (as we shall discuss later).
Experiencing refers to both the individual and group experiences
of staff members who work with particular kinds of trajectories;
these profoundly affect the ultimate control of a trajectory.

Diagnoses and Trajectory Schemes:
Their Contingencies and Complexities

Bringing the trajectory to as successful as possible an outcome, with a minimum of harm to the patient, requires identifying the source of the illness—that is, its diagnosis. *Diagnosing the illness* is the health worker's term for the beginning steps in trajectory work. Of course, the ill person will often have done work to manage the illness prior to seeking professional help, but for health workers the trajectory control begins with a diagnostic phase. After making a diagnosis, the physician has an imagery of what the trajectory shape will be, the kinds and degrees of hazard in each phase, the kinds of actions required to keep the patient on course, the resources and skills required to do so, and the anticipated contingencies that may cause the trajectory to go off course. He has also a plan to correct the altered course. In addition, the diagnostic phase includes both locating the patient's current position on the illness course, and estimating current and possible future dangers and risks. In our terms, a *trajectory scheme* is envisioned that involves an organization of tasks to keep the patient as safely as possible on course.

As a consequence of technological advances, the diagnostic process has become more rapid, efficient, and reliable. Yet a characteristic of contemporary diagnostic technology is that it gives an array of diagnostic options, whose results may range from very reliable to very questionable, be easy or difficult to carry out, require minimal to maximal skilled resources, vary in degree and kind of potential risks to the patient, and be inexpensive or very costly. A specific diagnostic procedure may possess varying combinations of these features. Also, the diagnostic process itself may require few or many methods, and be rapidly made or necessitate waiting for the disease progresssion before definitive diagnosis is possible.

Depending upon the illness, as well as on the patient's location on an extended illness course and the characteristics of the means of diagnosis, a physician must contend with different types of problems. Choices must be made not only on which diagnostic means to use but also on their combinations and sequences. When diagnosing breast tumors, for instance, biopsy, thermography, or mammography are available; for cardiac disorders there are electrocardiography, traditional chest x-ray, echocardiography, heart catheterization, along with an array of laboratory techniques. Choosing a means for diagnosis is further complicated by the weighing of potential risks associated with the technology against its reliability, and reliability against cost, and physician's legal safety against patient's clinical safety (Ingelfinger, 1978). Misbalancing or missequencing can occur; consequently, misdiagnosing and mislocating are possible. In part, these errors occur because the presenting symptoms may not match the actual severity of the illness, or a patient's expression of discomfort and distress may not match the phases anticipated by the diagnostic findings. Hence, vigorous diagnostic and locational procedures may be postponed. And, of course, for some illnesses the diagnosis can be very difficult.

In spite of the array of diagnostic approaches available today, a diagnostic search may encounter many problems, particularly in estimating the reliability of diagnostic means. Physicians may need to be careful in assessing the reliability since clinical laboratories, x-ray centers, and the like may vary in the quality of their work. A great deal of experience may be necessary to make reliable judgments. For example, an experienced oncologist remarked:

> I think you must learn to know who you can trust. Who overreads, who underreads. I have got x-rays all over town, so I've had the chance to do it. I know that when Schmidt at X hospital says, "There's a suspicion of a tumor in this chest," it doesn't mean much because she, like I, sees tumors everywhere. She looks under her bed at night to make sure there's not some cancer there. When Johns at the same institution reads it and says, "There's a suspicion of a tumor there," I take it damn seriously because if he thinks it's there, by God, it probably is. And you do this all over town. Who do you have confidence in and who none?

This illustration shows how cautious and even calculating a physician may need to be in assessing the quality of a diagnostic report and how useful it is to know the strengths and weaknesses of the diagnosticians and the diagnostic laboratories customarily relied upon. Diagnostic reliability is not foolproof. Physicians are increasingly at the mercy of the work of clinical laboratory technicians and other diagnostic technicians, whose reliability may not be easy to judge. Errors may arise also not only from misinterpretation but from machine error. Some machines have to be calibrated carefully or otherwise the test results that they produce can be inaccurate.

Complexity of Therapeutic Management

The complexity of organizing therapeutic action is due not only to the problematic character of many trajectories but also to the number, range, and organization of tasks involved in the therapeutic action. As mentioned earlier, when an illness is understood well, the standard operating procedures can readily control the trajectory. However, even relatively expectable trajectories can develop unanticipated complexities, especially around organizational issues. Moreover, just as modern medical technology offers more diagnostic options, there are now also more therapeutic options. Breast cancer, for example, can be treated with surgery, radiation, and chemotherapy; there are several types of each of those, and they can be used alone or in combination or in different combinations. The physician's choice is, of course, based on the type of cancer, its extent, and the reliability of available therapies. But the choice of therapy is also influenced by personal, medical, and social ideologies (sets of belief about certain kinds of surgery or drugs, convictions about womanhood and sexual relations), and the cost, convenience, available resources, and consideration of clinical safety.

Suppose that the trajectory goes off course, either from the unfolding of the illness itself or from unexpected contingencies, such as drug reaction, flare-up of another existing disease, or the development of a new disease from the therapy itself. In that event, then new therapeutic option decisions must be made.

Depending upon the given trajectory, these may be few or many, major or minor, as made throughout its various phases. Operational decisions must also be made. Option decisions may be initiated by the physician or other physicians, or suggested by a nurse, or initiated by the patient and family. With the increased strength of the patients' rights movement and the concern for "informed consent," the participation of patient and kin in option decision making becomes more crucial—especially if the options are risky or their potential psychological and biographical impacts are great.

Today, because of a larger number of extended unstable trajectories, the trajectories are characterized by multiple crucial "option points" (our term), where many personnel who have somewhat different stakes in the case may be weighing and pressing their respective views about various possible options. In large medical centers where problematic trajectories are most numerous, trajectory-oriented debates among health professionals are an ongoing occurrence—debates over trajectory location, diagnostic and therapeutic options, risks of the options, and the future shape of a given patient's trajectory.

Under the many illness conditions, trajectory management often shifts between or among various medical specialists. Even though one physician may be in charge throughout the total trajectory, as the problems and priorities change, various medical specialists may become major managers for a period of time, with the responsibility shifting from one to the other. Coordination of care may understandably be difficult when there are divergent views over options and priorities. Quite often the nurses, who function as integrators or coordinators of the many tasks entailed in the total diagnostic and therapeutic action, are caught in the middle of these diverse points of view. Their problems can become very difficult when the several specialists are not aware of each other's perspectives and so give conflicting medical orders.

To illustrate a highly complex and problematic trajectory, we shall present the case of Mrs. Price (Fagerhaugh and Strauss, 1977). This type of patient is all too familiar in acute care hospitals.

A Problematic Case

Mrs. Price, forty-five years old, was hospitalized for the fourth time. She had been diagnosed as having lupus erythematosus two years previously. During this period, both the treatment and the disease had drastically altered the quality of her life. For example, she could not engage in her one great pleasure, gardening, because sunlight exacerbated the lupus. As a result of her lupus, she had (1) pericarditis and (2) pleuritis, both of which caused pain; (3) cerebritis, which caused some personality change and a tendency toward tremors and convulsions; and (4) chronic obstructive lung disease from the lupus and her heavy smoking. As a result of steroid treatment to control the lupus, she further developed (5) a gastric ulcer for which surgery was required, and (6) cushinoid syndrome.

She was readmitted to the hospital because of continued chest pain. The lupus specialist suspected a pleuritic flare-up from the lupus and recommended hospitalization for reevaluation and a course of action to retard the illness process. She was readmitted to the same nursing unit where she had previously been a patient. During the previous hospitalization she was found to have a low tolerance for pain, which had resulted in drug dependency. The staff anticipated that pain management would be a problem.

During the first three days of hospitalization the house staff was busy evaluating her illness status; this involved innumerable blood studies, an electrocardiogram, and chest x-rays. On the second hospital day she could not be roused from sleep, so there was concern over extension of the cerebritis. Hence, an electroencephalogram was done. Meanwhile the patient was having increased chest pain, which the staff had difficulty controlling. On the seventh day she had increased abdominal pain—pain had developed three days earlier—but the early tests were negative. A number of possibilities were posed: bowel obstruction, extension of lupus, gastric ulcers secondary to the steroid drugs, or reaction to the heavy use of narcotics to control the pain. She also had an episode of sudden sharp chest pain. Another electrocardiogram was done, but the results were negative. Continuous intravenous infusions were started because she was developing fluid and electrolyte imbalance from the nausea and an inability to take food. The house staff decided that gastric suction would relieve her continued nausea and discomfort. She pulled out the gastric tube because she could not tolerate the gagging caused by the tube. Antinausea drugs were added to the drug list. Then a gastrointestinal specialist was consulted about her abdominal pain and nausea. Further blood and gastric studies were done.

On the fourteenth day a definitive diagnosis was made: she had developed a huge gastric ulcer. Also a chest x-ray showed a broken rib. Both were attributed to the steroid, yet the staff dared not stop the drug because the lupus would then get out of control. Everyone was upset by this new development, as well as by the continued deterioration of the patient's condition.

Immediate treatment problems were posed. The medical choices were limited. In the patient's current physical state she was a poor surgical risk. Yet the size and location of the ulcer, unless immediately treated, had dangerous consequences; there could be erosion and hemorrhage and/or peritonitis, or it could cause pancreatitis, both potentially fatal or at least extremely painful.

Numerous specialists were consulted. After much debate the decision was made to radiate her stomach to knock out the acid-producing cells and thus prevent further extension of the ulcer. The radiation dosage would be kept low so that other organs (particularly the kidney, which can become involved from the lupus itself) would not be compromised. She would be given a series of twelve radiation treatments extending over fifteen days. Concurrently, continuous hyperalimentation treatments were started to overcome the malnutrition. The physicians explained to the patient the limited choices, why the treatments were necessary, and that the radiation dosage would be extremely low. Mrs. Price agreed reluctantly because she was very frightened of radiation. A respiratory specialist was consulted regarding the rib fracture; a decison was made not to vigorously treat the fracture.

In the ensuing twelve days, her nausea increased and she

had several days of diarrhea, both related to the radiation. She would frequently resist the treatment, either because she felt too ill or because she doubted the wisdom of the therapy. On some days she could be persuaded by the staff, but increasingly she resisted. Or she would agree in the morning but change her mind in the afternoon. Finally, the staff in desperation gave her intravenous tranquilizers prior to the treatment to make her sleepy and less resistant.

Over the weeks, numerous specialists streamed in and out, but with no one person coordinating the care. After a number of episodes where the many doctors would write conflicting medical orders, the house staff pushed for a discussion about who should coordinate the care. A decision was reached; house staff and the gastrointestinal specialist together would be the major coordinators, and all new medical orders issued by attending staff would be discussed first with the house staff. The nursing staff sighed in relief because at least the ''mess'' would be under control. However, the coordination of effort continued to break down from time to time. One physician in particular would telephone the nursing desk with orders based on his past experience with the patient. This created much tension within the house medical staff.

Blood studies next indicated a low hemoglobin count. Blood transfusions were given. The nurses were becoming increasingly weary of the daily hassles with the patient, who wished to delay the various treatments.

On the twenty-seventh day she developed tremors of the hands and legs. She became very anxious since she saw this as a possible forerunner to convulsions. Because of her great anxiety, the staff had difficulty making an assessment of her actual condition, so they took a stance of ''wait and see.'' Mrs. Price thought immediate action was called for and again phoned her attending physician, who ordered drugs without consulting the house staff. Of course, this angered them. Mrs. Price's tremors did subside a few days later.

Because of continued nausea, all drugs—some thirty a day—were administered by injection. Since the injection sites were becoming fibrous knots, the nurses were concerned not only about the poor drug absorption but also about the possibility of infection because of the high steroid dose.

On the thirtieth day she developed joint pains and swelling of hands, elbows, feet, and knees—all symptoms of lupus. Steroid drug dosage was adjusted. In a few days the symptoms subsided.

On the thirty-third day the radiation treatments were completed. The patient had gained weight from the hyperalimentation treatment. A few days later the hyperalimentation was stopped since she was less nauseated and had less abdominal pain. A decision was made to reevaluate the results of the radiation treatment by x-ray after another week. The staff were hopeful that the radiation would be effective. A pulmonary function test was done, and a decision was made to start pulmonary treatment using an intermittent-positive-pressure respiratory machine and postural drainage for her chronic lung disease. However, the respiratory treatments were irregularly done because the patient found the treatments painful for she suffered broken ribs.

On the forty-first day the x-rays showed no decrease in her ulcer's size. Further gastric studies showed no appreciable decrease in gastric secretions. There was much troubled discussion among the staff. Mrs. Price was blamed for her uncooperativeness in taking antacids to prevent the ulcers and her continued chain smoking, which increased the gastric secretions. The patient, of course, was very upset. She commented to the researcher, "I knew all along the radiation wouldn't work. All I probably got out of the radiation is kidney damage."

During the next few days there was much discussion among a number of specialists about the next course of treatment. A decision was reached; the only alternative was a subtotal or total gastric resection. There were surgical risks, but without this intervention the consequences would be great. With the surgery she might live for several more years. So she was informed of the recommendation. The staff realized that her decision to accept surgery would be a difficult one.

For the next three weeks she agonized over whether or not to have the surgery. Her husband thought it was the only alternative. The psychiatrist thought that the patient, if discharged without surgery, would "drive the husband crazy," and that she would not consent to a nursing home. So surgery, the staff reasoned, should be done.

During this period the patient talked about dying to her husband, the psychiatrist, and the social researcher. The three discussed among themselves her sad dilemma and how they could help her. The staff now had difficulty in talking about dying with her as well as in interacting with her. She frequently stated that having been saved from death twice, she didn't know if she wanted to be saved again. She would take her chances without surgery and so hemorrhage and die. She was weary of all the uncertainty and pain. She was also talking more about wanting to commit suicide. The psychiatrist consulted with a suicide expert who thought the probability of her seriously considering suicide was low. Still the staff could not dismiss this possibility. As a precaution, her clothes were taken home, and money and drugs were removed from her purse, because she was talking about taking a taxi and jumping off the bridge.

On the sixty-seventh day the x-rays showed an increase in the size of the ulcer. There was total agreement among the physicians, including the psychiatrist, that a gastrectomy was required and should occur while the lupus was stable. For the next seven days she agonized over whether to have the gastrectomy. The physicians tried to answer the many questions as best they could. She was encouraged to consult other specialists and did so. They all agreed that a gastrectomy was essential. Her husband backed them. A relative persuaded her the surgery would be essential. She finally signed the consent for surgery. She was transferred to a gastrointestinal surgical unit. The surgery was successful, and Mrs. Price was weaned finally from the pain-controlling narcotics, but not without considerable interactional difficulties between the staff and her. Indeed, the purely physiological (surgical-pain trajectory) orientation of the surgical staff maximized the interactional problems. After 112 days, she was discharged, free of her ulcers but still having to live with her lupus.

This case illustrates the numerous difficulties encountered in keeping the patient's illness under control. The difficulties stem from (1) the multiple illness trajectories; (2) the multiple trajectory managers and the confusion over coordination of their efforts to control the trajectory; (3) the uncertainty surrounding therapeutic interventions; (4) the numerous unexpected contingencies; (5) the patient's active participation in the therapeutic actions and decisions, which ran counter to the staff's concerns and efforts; and, finally, (6) the cumulative impact on all parties concerned—the patient, staff, and kin. As noted earlier, given the complexity of such trajectories, the trajectories are not managed in the usual medical-nursing sense; they can be managed to some degree, but more accurately speaking they are really shaped and experienced. We should add that the case of Mrs. Price was complicated further because of chronic pain and issues of "dying," a common situation in acute care hospitals today. Issues of risk and danger color every phase of this patient's trajectory.

Safety and Trajectory Work

Now that we have sketched the complexity of trajectory management, we turn to the actual work involved in this management.

Tasks: Cluster, Sequence, and Organization. Work as commonly defined involves effort, tasks, and a goal: the *Random House Unabridged Dictionary* (1966) characterizes it as "exertion or effort directed to produce or accomplish something . . . something to be made or done; a task or undertaking." A useful way to analyze the work of managing even an unproblematic trajectory is to think of it as involving clusters of tasks (Hughes, 1971). There are many such clusters that must be simultaneously and/or sequentially carried out, but errors and failures can occur at any point in doing them and necessitate additional corrective tasks. Moreover, clinical safety work requires not only purely medical and technical clusters of tasks but also the organizational underpinning of countless tasks done by other workers, so that a minimum of harm is done to the patient.

As noted earlier, a trajectory extends over time and possesses phases around which physicians and nurses develop a trajectory scheme. Involved in that are many types of work to keep the trajectory on course. We shall refer to the staff's visualization of their total work for a given trajectory, over time, as the *arc of work*. This arc includes work done during all the trajectory phases and miniphases. In the more routine diseases, this visualized arc of work may be quite precise. In problematic trajectories, envisioning it is much less precise. Regardless of degree of preciseness during each phase, various decisions are made that certain actions should be taken; for instance, to monitor the cardiovascular system, get another x-ray, continue or discontinue a drug. The point at which different actions must be taken we shall call *trajectory option points*. The term is apt because, at each option point, there are choices about different clusters of tasks that must be ordered sequentially or simultaneously in order to complete the tasks. If there are defects in the organizational arrangements, then there will be a corresponding difficulty in following the sequence and the timing necessary for the next task. The requisite organizational resource base may include proper skills, sufficient personnel, drugs, equipment, enough time, and so on. While some of these resources may be located on the unit itself, others may need to come from other departments, or even from outside the hospital (for instance, machine repair). Ordinarily physicians do not concern themselves with the operational details of task accomplishment. The supervision and articulation of various tasks usually falls within the provinces of nurses and various technicians.

While an x-ray technician or laboratory technician focuses only on the immediate tasks of taking an x-ray or drawing blood and generally is not concerned about trajectory considerations, the physician and nurse are at least implicitly focused on those considerations as well as on the obvious work. At a particular moment, a specific task may absorb the physician's and the nurse's attention, but the patient's trajectory phase and location on a hazardous course are rarely, if ever, forgotten.

Types of Safety Tasks. In getting a given task completed with efficiency and with a minimum of clinical harm, the task structure will call for carrying out bundles of tasks that pertain to the various dangers and risks associated with them. However, each of these pertains to one or another of the following types of tasks. (Consideration of them will be central to the discussion throughout this book.) First of all, there are safety tasks related to medical-nursing technical matters (diagnosis, therapy, and palliative): that is, clinical safety tasks. These loom very large because of the high numbers of unstable trajectories and the many hazards associated with them. Second, since the patient participates (unless unconscious) in various clinical tasks, then fear and anxiety, or untimely or inappropriate interactions of personnel with the patient, or neglect of personnel to make explicit the patient's task can wound sensibilities and even self-esteem, as well as have consequences for clinical safety. Thus, there also are tasks that pertain to identity safety: that is, tasks involving staff interactions with patients to assure that self-esteem and sensibilities are not damaged. Third, and related to the above, there are other tasks concerned with bodily comfort safety: that is, with managing discomforts and pains associated with position and movement, with various discomforting bodily reactions, or with inflicted pain or discomfort generated by treatments. Fourth, both patient and staff must maintain their respective composure safety in order to do necessary tasks. Loss of composure can upset the smooth completion of a task or even be hazardous. Finally, because certain task structures involve bundles of tasks done by many workers, their work often calls for coordination of these—which are both sequentially and simultaneously ordered—along with resources necessary to do the tasks. In short, articulation safety work is necessary to avoid the mistiming and misorganization of the task structure.

In addition, work with kin may be called for. The personnel may need to explain the necessity of a given procedure or assist kin in maintaining composure. But the kin, like the patient, also participate in trajectory management. They too assess, monitor, prevent, and rectify potential dangers and risks as the trajectory unfolds. Here is a dramatic example: a father was anxiously accompanying his young, sedated son who was being wheeled out of his room to the surgical theater. The boy began to choke because his tongue was blocking his windpipe. The father—skilled at first aid procedures—quickly grabbed the tongue and pulled it free.

In sum, in order that a given task be carried out efficiently and with a minimum of harm, safety tasks are executed that relate to clinical safety, identity safety, bodily comfort safety, composure safety, and articulation safety. Not only are these integral components of the total task structure but they may also be differentially important at different phases and miniphases of the trajectory. Their importance for both task structure and trajectory phases will vary according to the following: the number and kind of resources required; the degree and kind of potential dangers and risks that must be assessed, prevented, monitored, minimized, and rectified; and the amount of patient and kin participation required. As will be evident in the next chapter, all of these safety task components must be sequentially and simultaneously ordered along the entire trajectory.

In different trajectory phases and at different places of work, different patterns of safety work can be observed. For instance, during the preoperative phase of a surgical trajectory, clinical safety tasks loom large because the staff must assess, prevent, and minimize potential risks associated with the impending surgery. Concurrently, safety tasks related to the patient's body comfort, identity, and composure are very necessary. During surgery itself, the risks can be numerous, so there is an exquisite ordering of the many clinical tasks that involve highly skilled personnel and other resources. More often than not, patients are unconscious, so psychosocial work is not necessary. Later in the recovery room, clinical safety tasks continue to be important, because the primary focus is on returning the patient's body to proper physiological functioning following the surgical trauma and the effects of anesthesia. Identity safety is usually of minimum concern here since the patient is actually or nearly unconscious. Once back on the unit, during the next days in the postoperative phase, clinical safety and body comfort safety tasks continue to be important, because the patient is recovering from the surgical trauma as well as from various medical and nursing interventions necessary to keep the trajectory on course. However, since the patient is reacting and many tasks require his or her participation, it follows that composure and identity work with patients looms very large for the staff.

A notable feature of safety work, particularly for nurses, is the fusion of many task clusters whose several safety concerns are part of the task structure. The sequencing of tasks within a task cluster may be routinized or flexible depending upon its miniphases. Field observations on a cardiac surgical recovery unit illustrate these points:

> I watched Nurse T. working today about an hour. In general the work was mixed. She changed the blood transfusion bottle. She milked the tubing to take out the air bubble. Later she changed the tubing again. She drew blood and placed the blood in test tubes for tests. She milked the urine tube once. She took a temperature. She put a drug injection into the tube leading to the patient's neck. She added potassium solution to the non-automated IV. But all the while she had in focus, although not necessarily glancing directly at it, the screen which registered the heart action. She punched the computer button to get the fifteen minute readout of cardiac functioning. She later milked the tube leading from the patient's chest. Periodically she marked down both the reading and some of what she had observed and done. Once the patient stirred. As she touched his arm, she said quite nicely that she was about to give him an injection that would relax him. He indicated he heard. Another time she noticed him stirring and switched off the light above him, saying to him, "That's better, isn't it?" At one point she assessed the blood pressure was not dropping rapidly enough. She tells the resident, suggesting he do something. He hesitates, but she keeps nudging until he goes into action.

In this sequence of tasks, which will be repeated over and over again throughout the following hours, we see the nurse's focus on matters of safety, comfort, and even the patient's psychological state, as she monitors, records, and assesses various aspects of the clinical condition of the patient. Mistiming and misorganization of a task structure are not uncommon, since many departments involved in carrying out many chains of tasks must be coordinated; yet the task sequencing can go awry because of many departmental contingencies. When an unexpected contingency or an error delays the task sequence, then the consequences may disturb the trajectory phase progression. They may also wound a patient's sensibilities and may produce or increase bodily discomfort. The contingencies or errors can even lead to potential or actual death. The former happened to an alert and experienced patient who during a prolonged wait outside the x-ray room on a gurney, with only the transport worker in attendance, barely saved himself by insisting on his return to the ward for a saving medication.

Case Illustration: Bodily Comfort Safety. Another case example will serve to illustrate not only the several types of safety tasks but also their necessary sequencing. It also makes vivid how mistiming and misorganization can delay the tasks.

An eighty-year-old lady was hospitalized for very severe back pain that was diagnosed as a ruptured lumbar disc. Eventually it was relieved by a combination of medications and the use of an electric cutaneous stimulator. After two days of using various combinations of analgesic drugs and heat, her severe pain noticeably decreased, and she was able to eat some food. However, the coaxial tomography (CAT) scan necessary for diagnosing the location and degree of lumbar disc damage was delayed, because of the heavy demands on this particular diagnostic department.

The nurses gave a pain medication prior to her finally undergoing the CAT scan test. They did this to minimize the pain and discomfort associated with moving her (to and from the bed-gurney-CAT scan table). The transport worker and the nurses worked together when moving the patient from bed to gurney, so that her pain might be minimized. Unfortunately, the patient was very sensitive to becoming cold, for that aggravated her back pain. Although the nurses realized that her getting cold would increase her pain, they forgot to add extra blankets.

Unexpectedly, outside of the CAT room there was a considerable delay, for another patient had received a higher priority because his case was of an emergency nature. But the elderly lady, while waiting a full hour in the drafty hallway because the patient area was crowded with other patients whose schedules were also delayed by the emergency case, became very cold. So again she developed severe back pain. Her daughter, who had accompanied her, finally located an unidentified hospital worker and requested some blankets. Because of the delay, the scan was rescheduled for later in the afternoon. The elderly lady, now in considerable pain, was transported back to her bed.

Then the nurses rushed into the breach with pain medications and a heating pad. Immediately thereafter dinner was served, but because the patient was in great pain she could not eat. And directly after the food's delivery, the transport man came with a gurney. The daughter asked him to "hold off for a while" until her mother felt better. Once the pain became less severe, the patient was moved again to the gurney, but now she was covered with extra blankets. Then the daughter, mother, and transport worker made the trip together to the CAT equipment.

The scan test, however, involved moving the patient onto the scan table. A technician who was to do the scanning explained what was to occur during the test and emphasized the importance of not moving so as to obtain a successful test. Then he carried out the many tasks related to the test, concurrently offering encouraging statements and asking the patient, "Are you all right?" Meanwhile, the daughter talked to her to distract her, also making encouraging statements.

The scanning finished, the technician telephoned the transport department to have the patient moved back to her room. However, since fewer transport personnel were on the evening shift, there was another delay. Again the patient was kept waiting. Finally the daughter cajoled another technician into moving her mother. Once back in bed, the mother commented that although she was steadily feeling more comfortable, she was now only back to where she had started.

Among the phenomena that this case illustrates are the unforeseen contingencies that can delay completion of the planned work. There was a failure of comfort safety (keeping the patient warm), which thereby decreased effective management of the pain (previously that management had been relatively successful). Despite failure to keep the patient warm, the nurses attempted to coordinate the analgesics and the patient's movements in order to minimize her bodily discomfort and pain. The unexpected contingencies at the radiology department, however, limited how much the nurses could control the pain. Also in this case the kin's work partly compensated for organizational lapses. This type of work tends not to be recognized by the staff. In general, such a lengthening of diagnostic task structure as seen in this case is not uncommon, because of the increased number of diagnostic services in hospitals today and the difficulties of articulating ward work with their work. Moreover, here the lengthening of task structure involved not only this particular patient but others whose schedules were upset by the unexpected contingency at the CAT department.

Perhaps most important, this case illustrates the finite resources available at the hospital, as well as the competition among patients and among departments for those resources. This patient was ''bumped'' to a lower priority by an emergency patient who had a higher priority because of his dangerous state, thereby disarticulating the anticipated task sequence. To keep groups of patients on course, an immense amount of safety work is necessary, and this results in much implicit competition for resources among patients. The expected contingencies, together with the finite resources, shape not only the task sequences but also contribute to shaping the patients' trajectories and so, too, their safety.

Summary

By considering safety with respect to an illness trajectory, one can begin to focus on the complex organizational and work arrangements and staff-staff and patient-staff interactions that must be organized in order to assure safe patient care. Yet the uncertainties of both the illnesses themselves and the effects of medical technologies, plus the many unexpected contingencies, create disruptions that contribute to shaping the illness course. Staff must make difficult decisions frequently throughout the entire course of an illness. Safety requires the alignment of clinical, identity, bodily comfort, composure, and articulation safety tasks. These may constitute important work in and of themselves at various phases of the evolving illness but also may be components of an overall task (as would be the case in clinical work). These safety tasks often occur simultaneously and shift constantly throughout the illness trajectory.

3

∽◠∽

Identifying the Complex Sources
of Clinical Hazards

The first concern in patient care by health professionals is the patient's clinical safety as related to technical matters of diagnosis, treatment, and palliation of disease. Their clinical safety work includes several major work processes, which will be discussed in the remainder of this book. The processes are (1) assessing the many potential sources of hazards; (2) preventing and (3) monitoring them; (4) minimizing the necessary risks inflicted by staff members when attempting to reverse the patient's illness course; and (5) rectifying hazards once they occur because of malfunctioning, error, or other unexpected contingencies. Depending upon various phases of a trajectory and in different workplaces, varied importance will be placed on one or more aspects of these work processes. However, virtually all clinical actions involve aspects of each.

Recollect that clinical safety looms large because the more that devices, including various types of equipment, are used in care and the more complicated they are, the greater is their likelihood of failure. When used with patients in highly acute, unstable, and problematic illness states, control of the hazards becomes increasingly difficult. In the technical literature, health professionals' concerns about clinical safety are usually discussed in terms of preventing and managing iatrogenic illness, with the greatest effort being directed at identifying the causes of technology-related iatrogenic illnesses. Patients with these illnesses are concentrated in intensive care units where the number

53

of medical devices are also greatest (Abramson, Wald, Grenvik, and Snyder, 1980; Agarwal, 1980; Couch, Tilney, Rayner, and Moore, 1981; Murray, 1981; Steel, Gertman, Crescenzi, and Anderson, 1981).

Thus, Steel, Gertman, Crescenzi, and Anderson (1981), in a study of adverse occurrences in a tertiary care university hospital, found that 35 percent of adverse effects were related to the use of medical devices, and 42 percent were related to drug use. And Shepherd (1983) concluded that improper design, selection, application, maintenance, and utilization of medical devices contributed to their failures. Likewise, Abramson, Wald, Grenvik, and Snyder (1980), in a five-year study of a general medical-surgical intensive care unit, found that human error contributed to the 145 injurious incidents to patients. Misuse of medical devices accounted for 30 percent of the occurrences, while communication error and nurse understaffing accounted for 34 percent. Abramson's study also showed a pattern of high incidence of error associated with the seasonal influx of inexperienced physicians and nurses. Similarly, Shepherd's (1983) study of malfunctioning medical devices reported that 38 percent were due to "educational deficiencies" and 39 percent to "equipment misuse."

Since proficiency of staff is inversely related to the frequency of iatrogenic occurrences, the proper training of professionals with respect to these is increasingly deemed very important. However, the lag between technological innovation and the clinically skilled abilities to manage the risks associated with that technology has been a perennial problem in health care. As well-trained and experienced as staff may be, and even though they try to anticipate potential hazards and build mechanisms to manage them before a new technology is used, there are always unexpected risks. (This is an important point to understand; otherwise, staffs may get misjudged for not assuring more safety than, in fact, they can.) An extended amount of time is needed for working with and "experiencing" a new technology and "getting the bugs out"—so as to specify its potential hazards as well as the necessary skills and resources for managing them. In most cases, institutional arrangements and formal education programs for assuring clinical safety occur after rather than before a period of technology usage.

It has been estimated that one million medical injuries occur annually; of these 200,000 involve some negligence (Trandel-Korenchuk and Trandel-Korenchuk, 1983). Over the years, medical malpractice actions have steadily increased, costing nearly a billion dollars a year. One of every nine malpractice claims involved a medical device, and these had the highest average indemnity. Then, too, under the Hospital Corporate Liability ruling (the Darling decision), not only the physicians and hospital administrators but also the nurses and other health care practitioners are liable for clinical negligence (Duran, 1980; Leonard, 1983). The nursing profession's drive toward more professional autonomy also means that nurses are personally liable for practically everything they do (Duran, 1980).

The difficulties encountered in assuring clinical safety are due in part to the multiple sources of hazard and their complex interactions. Moreover, safety rests on complex coordination of hospital support services that are concerned with selecting, maintaining, and distributing medical devices. Thus, any organizational contingencies that disrupt this coordination can disrupt clinical safety. In light of these considerations, we shall first discuss the sources and dimensions of hazards, and their interactions, as they affect clinical safety. Then we shall discuss the varieties of safety tasks engaged in by professionals that must be coordinated when controlling the many sources of hazard. This will be followed by a discussion of the immense amount of work involved as well as the problems encountered in the selection and maintenance of medical machines and devices.

Hazard: Sources, Dimensions, Profiles, and Source Interaction

The matching of safety resources and the organization of work for assuring safety are usually based on a consideration of the potential sources and dimensions of hazards.

Consider first the several sources of hazards. Perhaps the most obvious source is the illness itself and the patient's bodily responses. However, the patient's behavior can also be a source of hazard, if the patient does not "cooperate"—refuses a necessary treatment, does not remain immobile during a potentially dangerous procedure, pulls out tubes from various body orifices, or fiddles with the dials on a machine. Also, the drugs, machinery, and procedures themselves are all potential sources of hazard. Workers, too, may be a source because they lack proper skills or make errors or become tired. The hospital's highly technologized environment can be a source: improper wiring, crowded space, high noise level, and so on. Finally, there are the possibilities of institutional misarrangement or nonarrangements that can become sources of hazard.

There are several important dimensions of hazard. Each dimension ranges along a continuum from low to high and may shift in importance at given phases of a given trajectory. Let us now elaborate the meanings of the terms used for the various dimensions:

- *Number, rate of occurrence,* and *duration* refer respectively to the total number, how often they occur, and how long they last.
- *Gravity* refers to the degree and extent of the danger or risk. Moreover, a risk may be a threat only to the patient, to both staff and patient, or may extend to the total ward and even to the hospital. (For example, an electrical short from a machine may be hazardous to the patient or to the staff, or in varying combinations to patient, staff, and machinery, or can be a source of explosions and fire that may extend to the total ward and even the entire hospital.)
- *Specificity* refers to the degree to which danger or risk can be explicitly identified as to its causes.
- *Predictability* is related to specificity. That is, the indicators and conditions for probable danger or risk are well known and readily anticipated.
- *Controllability* is the degree to which a hazard can be prevented and managed. That may range from easy to difficult, depending on the kinds of skills, resources, and speed of action required.
- *Rectifiability* is the extent to which hazards can be corrected,

whether from the progression of a danger or risk or from an error made by the staff, or from equipment malfunctioning. Some hazards cannot be rectified beyond a certain point. Others can be rectified within a specific time period or only at great cost of time or money.

An essential feature of these hazard dimensions is their variability over time. Quite often the knowledge gained through a period of practice, experience, and even error may be necessary before specificity, predictability, controllability, and rectifiability can be assured. Of course, new medical knowledge or a technological breakthrough may alter these salient dimensions.

The several sources of hazard vary in combination, and in association, with the hazard dimensions—as well as the different illnesses and their phases. For instance, the patient as a body system may be seriously though not gravely in danger. A potential danger from the illness itself then, as well as the risks associated with various medical measures done during the various phases of care, can be specified and predicted and controlled. In other illness conditions, however, the body system may not be immediately endangered; but in some miniphases the danger, or risks to it, as during a heart catheterization, may be quite high. The patient's behavior can also vary as a source of hazard. High anxiety, fear, or mental confusion may prevent a patient from participating in hazard minimization, or cause him or her to increase the potential riskiness of therapeutic or diagnostic procedures. Then, too, estimating a patient's behavior as a source of hazard on any of its various dimensions may be extremely difficult, as with a suicidal person. Also, diagnostic, palliative, and therapeutic measures that involve various machinery, procedures, and drugs will vary widely in the matter of danger or risk.

Because of all these variables, it is analytically possible to develop potential hazard profiles for the phases and miniphases of various trajectories. Actually, the staff now does this kind of assessing and locating but does so implicitly. Exhibit 1 shows one form that could be used to diagram a patient's potential hazard profile. Systematic use of such a profile may be useful

Exhibit 1. Patient Potential Hazard Profile.

	Potential Sources of Hazard					
Danger Risk Dimensions	*Patient's Illness*	*Patient's Behavior*	*Diagnostic/Palliative Therapeutic Sources*	*Personnel*	*Physical Environment*	*Institutional Arrangements*
Gravity High Low						
Specificity Unknown Known						
Predictability Difficult Easy						
Controllability Difficult Easy						
Duration Long Short						

for explicitly assessing hazards for particular patients. For instance, if a profile for Mrs. Price (see the previous chapter) were diagrammed, it would indicate, to begin with, someone who was gravely ill because of a breakdown of several body systems. To predict and control her continuing deterioration would be very difficult. Also, her behavior would be a constant source of risk because of her smoking, her not "cooperating" with treatments, and her "suicidal potential." Likewise, the staff's palliative interventions over the many days unfortunately might (and did) fall within an unfavorable range of the hazard dimensions. (The many specialists coming into and out of her care also added to the potential and unpredictable hazard.) In essence, Mrs. Price's profile indicated multidetermined hazards with many accompanying ambiguities and the successful outcome from the various interventions possibly very low unless managed with special planning. A profile explicitly diagrammed might have improved her care and prevented some of the staff's anger and extreme frustration.

Professionals do indeed take into account these hazard dimensions when making their assessments, since the dimensions determine the extent of preventing, monitoring, and rectifying required for maximizing clinical safety. For instance, if a procedure has known risks that are low in gravity, involve clear bodily indicators, and can be readily prevented, and the risks are both controllable once they occur and of short duration, then managing the risks is easy. The focus will be directly on the prevention of risk. By contrast, suppose that a given risk is high in gravity, its cause is multidetermined, the predictability of its occurrence and its control depend upon many kinds of information (patient reaction, laboratory tests, monitoring machine readouts, and so on)—then extensive monitoring and reassessing are required. Also necessary are experienced personnel who possess manipulative, observational, and interpretive skills. Risk priorities and the allocation of resources, in short, are based on such assessments.

Our concept of hazard profile is in keeping with current medical and nursing practice. For instance, under the approach used in carrying out "nursing process" (Gordon, 1976), assessment of the patient's physical and psychosocial status is first determined, to be followed by the identification of various associated physical or psychological "problems." Restated in safety language, such a "problem" is the identification of "what is at risk." This raises two questions: To what degree is there risk, and what is necessary to decrease or reverse it, based on which of its aspects are preventable, controllable, and rectifiable? To think this way should assist both in establishing priorities of risks and in establishing the frequency and degrees of assessing, monitoring, and rectifying the work required for controlling the risks.

Examination of articles or textbooks (whether nursing or medical) related to clinical care of patients reveals that care is always discussed in terms of what is abnormal, why it is abnormal, how much damage is involved, and how these are determined; what and why certain interventions are appropriate or inappropriate for the abnormal condition; what kinds of hazards there are and why certain ones are associated with the interventions; how to identify the hazards; what are the safety limits, how to determine them, and how to rectify them when hazards exceed the safety limit; and, finally, on what basis the effects of the interventions can be determined. The hazard profile perspective can sharpen the central concern that all professionals implicitly have when caring for patients: how to organize care to maximize safety and minimize harm.

A hazard profile as in Exhibit 1 takes into account only the sources of hazard and their dimensions. However, a more complex issue involved in clinical safety is anticipating how the sources of hazard interact and how instances of malfunctioning (procedural, technical, organizational), or an error that endangers one source, might impact on other sources. Maintenance of clinical safety involves anticipating this complex relationship, as diagrammed in Figure 1.

To illustrate the interactions in Figure 1, let us look at a common procedure: a vein cut-down for placing a needle or catheter in the vein, done in order to administer a drug by using a push pump. This intervention calls for a procedure to do the cut-down in order to place the needle or catheter into the

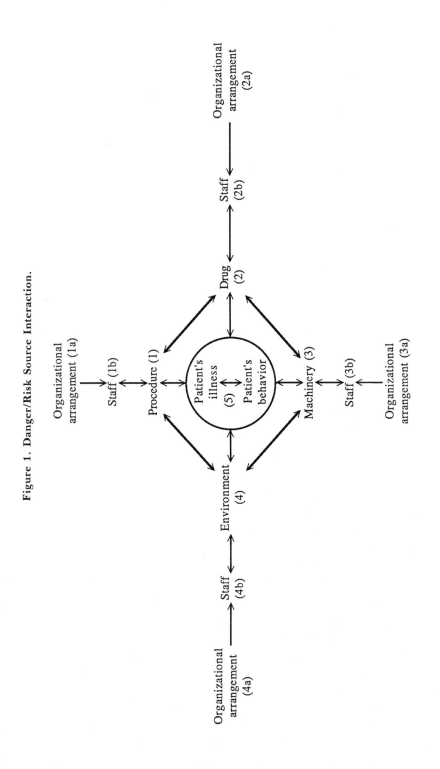

Figure 1. Danger/Risk Source Interaction.

patient's vein; a drug to be administered which is mixed into an intravenous solution bottle with tubing connected to the needle or catheter; connecting the tubing to the push pump; and environmental considerations, such as ensuring the availability of an electrical outlet to hook up the machine, making space arrangements for doing the cut-down procedure, placing the pump machine, and preparing the drug and intravenous materials. All of these actions can affect the patient both as a body system and as a person. The procedure, drug, pump, and environment all require organizational arrangements (1a, 2a, 3a, 4a) in order to procure safe and approved materials, and to prepare and maintain them. Thus an organizational misarrangement may negatively affect the task structure. Then, there are ward staff who attend to the safety requirements pertaining to the procedure of the cut-down, drug, machine, and environment (1b, 2b, 3b, 4b). Usually the ward staff involves two persons: a physician and a nurse. Staff must consider the overall safety of the intervention by anticipating the interaction of all four potential hazards, including themselves. A malfunctioning electrical outlet can lead to the pump not functioning, or shortcomings of space arrangements when doing the cut-down procedures can lead to the pump being knocked over. In preparing the drug, the correct dilution in the mixing of the drug must be taken into account, but also the solution used must be compatible with the drug. Also, the kind of drug used and the condition of the patient's veins must be considered when choosing what kind and size of needle or cannula to use. The rate of the drug administration must take into account both the condition of the patient and the kind of drug used.

So, we can imagine that the errors or malfunctions arising from any source (staff, environment, procedure, drug, machinery) can impact differentially on each source, and certainly on the patient. Also, the latter as a source of hazard—both the illness and the behavior of the patient—can negatively affect procedural safety. Once a patient is connected, possible risks of drug action in terms of the particular illness and danger state must be anticipated. In addition, the risks of drug action are related to the rate of drug administration, the pressure applied by the pump machine, and the viscosity of the drug. The patient's illness state—which might compromise the drug therapy—must be taken into account when setting the machine pressure and rate. Thus, clinical safety involves anticipating the complex interaction of procedure-drug-machine-patient, as well as how each malfunctioning or error in one source might affect another and so affect the total interaction. Of course, the complexity of interaction will vary with the complexities of the procedures and drugs, the illness statuses of patients, and the numbers of other medical measures used.

Characteristically, in acute care hospitals many kinds of drugs, procedures and machines are used simultaneously and in tandem. Hence there are risks associated with interactions of drug-drug, machine-machine, machine-environment, illness-illness, procedures-machines, for they all relate to clinical safety. Thus, a complex process of assessing, preventing, monitoring, minimizing, and rectifying multiple hazards that flow from these interactions are all required. In addition, these hazards must be given priority in terms of their danger/risk dimensions.

Clinical safety initially involves trying to map out the patient's hazard profile (that term and the associated chart, of course, are our inventions) for the various phases and miniphases of an anticipated trajectory. Indeed, clinical care protocols might be seen as a laying out of the expected safety work in terms of that detailed profile. One striking feature of contemporary acute care hospitals consists of the rapid changes in hazard profiles that evolve over the various phases of their patients' trajectories. The changes result, of course, from the clinical technology itself, plus the predominance of patients with highly unstable states of chronic illnesses. The huge armamentarium of means used to stabilize and reverse illness courses means that many clinical actions are rapidly applied, despite their potential risks. However, not only are there high-risk phases during the trajectory miniphases, but the items of danger/risk are constantly changing.

Both the foregoing hazard profile chart and the discussion of the sources of hazard interaction suggest that, within the hospital, different work sites will have characteristically different patterns of hazard profiles. In intensive care units, the potential dangers and risks are at a maximum, but there are variations of hazard within the various types of ICUs. For example, neonatal ICUs, as compared to adult ICUs, have extremely fragile patients whose bodies allow a smaller margin of error, so a major safety concern is with rectifiability done within a restricted time period. More important, neonatal ICUs represent a relatively new clinical area; this means that the dimensions (specificity, predictability, and so on) of many risks associated with the therapeutic actions are very high (Blackburn 1982). Diagnostic units, such as x-ray, pulmonary function laboratories, and heart catheterization laboratories, have very different hazard profiles. Likewise, nursing care units, such as neurosurgical units, as compared to rehabilitation nursing units, have vastly different profiles from one another.

Of concern to health professionals also are the cumulative effects arising from the source of danger/risk interactions. Thus, when multiple body systems are endangered—requiring the use of risky drugs, machines, and procedures—then an immense amount of clinical safety work is needed to prevent the danger/risk from getting out of hand. The cumulative effects include, as we have seen, not only the clinical hazards but may extend to the patients' and staff's composure, and then threaten their respective identities.

Here is an actual illustration of such a cumulative effect: without warning there is a failure of monitoring equipment hooked to a cardiac patient who is simultaneously receiving drugs via an intravenous push pump. The patient becomes very anxious and so becomes a source of further hazard. If the equipment failure cannot be quickly corrected—because of inadequate repair service or the absence of an experienced nurse who can usually be depended on for machine troubleshooting, or there is a lack of sufficient back-up machines—then risk to the patient is increased. This equipment failure can then involve the staff's composure and the identity safety of its members. In addition, that failure can disturb the composure of other patients. The ICU staffs' oft-used phrase "keeping your cool" is related to their maintaining their own composure in order to prevent potentially cumulative clinical risks.

Of current concern is the stress and burnout of nursing staff at acute hospitals, particularly those working in intensive care units (Graham, 1981; Maslach, 1976; Shubin, 1978). In the context of our discussion of hazards to staff composure and identities, this stress and burnout can be interpreted partly as a cumulative effect of those hazards. Likewise, the mental confusion termed "ICU psychosis" (Simon, 1980) and "coronary madness" (Schoenfeld, 1978), each affecting patients, might be viewed in terms of cumulative effects flowing from the many stresses found in a complicated, technologized environment.

Task Structure and Clinical Safety

As noted earlier, the anticipated risks associated with clinical actions must be operationalized by fashioning the necessary tasks into an organized task structure. Since risks are of varying numbers, kinds, and degrees, any given task structure will include safety requirements of various degrees and kinds. Those variations include:

> the diversity of their spatial and material properties
> the diversity of "clusters of tasks" that involve different types and levels of skilled health professionals, as well as different potential risks
> the degree of precision and speed of action required to order simultaneously and sequentially the cluster of tasks
> the degree of communication necessary among health professionals
> the degree of awareness that personnel must have of each other's safety jobs in the overall task structure
> the degree of flexibility in the temporal ordering of the task clusters
> the rectifiability arising from malfunctioning, error, or unexpected contingencies

In addition, a task structure often calls for a complex process of assessing, preventing, minimizing, monitoring, and rectifying potential risks. The component tasks must often be done by several personnel, either for effectiveness or because of necessity. To illustrate these points, here is a scene observed in a cardiac intensive care unit.

Mr. C., a patient in his late seventies, has serious congestive heart failure. He had been at the center of staff attention all morning. Considered the most seriously ill patient on the unit, he was placed in a room that directly faced the nursing station. The nurses described him as being irritable and anxious throughout the night.

The physicians had made a decision to insert a Swan-Ganz catheter to monitor his hemodynamic system more accurately. The nurses were anxious that the procedure be done soon because two new patients were scheduled for admission. However, the resident physician who was to do the procedure was not immediately available, as he was tied up with teaching rounds. Twice during the rounds, a nurse approached him to "get the show on the road" because of the impending admissions.

Since the work pace on the ward was slow and other patients were less seriously ill and were stabilized, there was an opportunity to provide "learning experiences" for a novice nurse. She was assigned to a task, assisted by several experienced nurses who were to tutor her. She brought the necessary equipment, machinery, and supplies to the bedside, following instructions in the procedure manual. A "crash cart" was also brought to the bedside. One of the nurses assisted her in setting up the machine and arranging the Swan-Ganz equipment. (This is a setup with some eleven tubes connected to various parts of the equipment, machine, and patient.) The assisting nurse indicated the various steps for doing this particular task—its do's and don't's, and the potential risks of error.

Another nurse calibrated a monitoring machine that would be connected to the patient, a very specialized monitor, custom-made to certain research requirements. Earlier, the head nurse had told me that because of its specialized nature, only a few nurses and technicians could fine-tune the machine. In fact, a few days earlier, when it required recalibration, a technician was contacted to correct the problem. This technician was unfamiliar with the machine, however, so could not correct the problem. Finally, the head nurse had to help in the recalibration.

The resident came, then, to insert the catheter. He explained to the patient again, as earlier that morning, that he would be putting a tube down through a neck vein. He said it was necessary to lie flat during the procedure, even though this might make breathing more difficult. An experienced nurse and the novice nurse both helped to position the patient. Then the physician and all the nurses donned masks.

In a nice manner, an experienced nurse informed the physician that there were two sets of sterile gloves, one for disinfecting the skin and the other for inserting the catheter. This nurse had told me earlier that she had insisted on a more elaborate, operating room type of setup for these kinds of procedures. Prior to her arrival on the unit there had been less strict aseptic techniques. Previous records showed a number of infections, but after more strict techniques were instituted, the infection rate had noticeably decreased.

While the physician was preparing himself and readying the equipment, another nurse came with a connection for the central monitor situated in the nursing station. The experienced nurse pointed out to the novice the proper connections and how they could be identified by the numbers of prongs and the color coding.

Then the physician disinfected the patient's skin in preparation for the procedure, but before doing so informed him that he would be cleansing the skin and that the solution would be cold. He asked the patient to lie still and to keep his hands out of the way. His task completed, the physician prepared the necessary equipment for the next steps in the procedure. Then he told the patient that his face would be covered with a towel. Throughout all of this, the novice nurse helped the physician, while the experienced nurse whispered information about both the next steps and the equipment that needed to be readied.

Shortly after the physician had prepared the patient, another experienced physician arrived to help. At the same time, yet another experienced physician, dressed in street clothes, stood at the doorway. The physicians exchanged information about the laboratory findings pertaining to this patient. They queried the resident about what he expected would be the pressure readings after putting down the catheter, given the patient's current condition. The resident speculated about that.

Before the experienced physician got into a sterile gown, he surveyed the situation and immediately removed a pillow from under the patient's head. The experienced nurse immediately caught the error that had been discovered and brought a rolled towel to place under the patient's neck. The physician explained to the resident why this position was preferred. The physician also asked the patient if he was "all right."

The resident anesthetized the vein cut-down area, assisted by the novice nurse. Before injecting the anesthetic, the resident told the patient that he would anesthetize the area and that some pricks would be felt. The nurse immediately moved over and held the patient's hand. The physician who was overseeing the procedure made suggestions to the resident about how to use the needle for getting better results. Giving this information was interspersed with telling the patient that he was "doing very well" and asking how he felt. Meanwhile, both nurses were looking at the monitoring machine.

The experienced doctor showed the resident how to locate the vein for incision and the best way to do it. The resident warned the patient that pressure would be felt but no pain. The physician gave low-voiced instructions to the resident. The procedure progressed nicely and relaxedly, with the resident even asking many technically related questions about cardiac management. While this was going on, the nurse remained with the patient, from time to time patting him, removing the towel to observe him, and informing him that "everything is fine." All the while she was glancing at the monitor.

The physician interrupted the resident's conversation, saying that the catheter had better be put in right away because there was danger of blood clotting if they dallied. He quickly prepared the catheter, then pushed it into the vein. The nurse immediately moved to the special monitor machine, making adjustments to it, writing on the paper readouts, and instructing the novice to prepare the various connections. Everybody looked at the monitor. The physician suggested that the catheter be pulled out "a tad," because the catheter position needed to be adjusted. Everybody watched the monitor for a while. A little later the physician informed the resident that everything had gone well and complimented the patient for being good. The physician and the resident exchanged technical information. Then the physician said he would leave the suturing to the resident. Meanwhile, both nurses helped the patient get comfortable. The more

experienced nurse discussed various critical points
about observation and care of the patient with the
novice.

This not unusal scene in a cardiac ICU suggests the complexity of the work done in achieving clinical safety. It illustrates
the various bundles of tasks that involve several personnel, and
that must be done sequentially and also organized simultaneously
into a task organization. First of all, the nurse assessed the potentially risky procedure in terms of the overall anticipated work
on the unit, because the procedural safety necessitated time and
personnel. After surveying the overall unit danger/risk level,
she trained a novice so that the latter could gain experience with
safety in risky procedures. In essence, as a member of the staff,
she was helping to build safety resources; the experienced physician was doing the same with the resident. Also, in readying
the necessary equipment, machinery, and supplies, as well as
doing the procedure, a back-up (crash cart, seasoned personnel) was made available to prevent and rectify possible risks
should anything go awry.

The physicians who were carrying out the procedure engaged in interaction with the patient so that he would not be
a source of danger and to maximize his composure safety. Also,
the physicians interacted with the patient before each minitask
that might endanger him. The nurse prevented the physician
from breaking aseptic technique, and this was done very tact-
fully so that his identity was not wounded.

Moreover, the personnel took into account various risk
potentials associated with the task phases. The physician entered
the scene when the risk potential was highest, taking over tasks
from the resident. Likewise, the experienced nurse took over
tasks from the novice when they required great skill, as with
the special monitor machine. In short, the experienced personnel engaged in monitoring and preventing those risks that might
be incurred by the actions of less experienced staff. When the
physicians were engaged in tasks that required much concen-
tration, the nurse took over composure-safety work with the
patient.

This case vignette also shows some consequences that can occur when various conditions are altered. As one can see, the consequences would have been different if (1) the number of seriously ill patients had been very high, (2) there had been a shortage of experienced nursing staff, (3) the experienced staff did not take into account the less-experienced staff's identity and composure safety, (4) the entire staff did not take into account the patient's identity and composure safety, (5) the tasks had been out of sequence, (6) the skills had not been matched with high-risk task phases, (7) there had been an unexpected breakdown of equipment and machinery, or (8) the patient's physical condition had changed. Different combinations of these conditions will, of course, have different consequences.

By contrast, the safety requirements are quite different in a cardiac resuscitation task structure. Then the patient is in a potentially grave physical state. There is a very short safety time limit from the time of observed danger and application of the resuscitation, and the procedure has many risks not only for the patient but for the staff as well. Similarly, consider the procedure to insert an intra-aortic balloon catheter (a tube, attached to a pump and with a sausage-shaped balloon on the tip, is inserted through an artery in the groin and passed into the aorta). This calls for a very specialized pump machine, special space, and teams of skilled personnel who work simultaneously and sequentially on different parts of a patient.

Generally, to manage the risks of patient care more efficiently, patients with similar trajectories and hazard profiles are grouped on the same ward. This enables a routinizing and patterning of the overall safety-task structure. The likelihood is then that fewer major task readjustments and reorganizations need be made if patients' hazard profiles do change. Hence, there is a strong drive for each specialty and subspeciality to have its own special unit, providing that hospital space and funds permit this. However, many problems are posed because of the present increase in problematic trajectories, combined with finite resources that do not permit an exact matching of resources to the danger/risk profiles, plus the multitude of organizational underpinnings on which task structure safety hinges.

Safety Considerations in Working with Machines

Throughout hospitals today, one sees vast amounts of medical equipment. Patients are cared for in electrically operated beds, often are hooked to many kinds of machines, and are taken to and from places where there is specialized machinery. Much of clinical safety, then, rests on the safety of the machines themselves and their associated software. In turn, this necessitates that a great deal of safety work be done by many levels of workers. Because of the varied properties of the machinery, this work is also highly varied. In general terms, machines have different functions—diagnosis, therapy, monitoring, relieving discomforts and pain, and substituting for an impaired body function. Thus, a partial list of properties of machines includes the following:

> function
> size
> cost
> numbers and kinds of models
> durability
> reliability
> new-old innovation
> servicing required
> skills, practice, and knowledge needed to set up the machine, connect it to the patient, and operate, monitor, and remove
> calibration required
> used alone or in conjunction with other machines
> numbers and kinds of supplies, drugs, and other software used with the machine
> external or internal to the body

Each of those properties has relevance to clinical safety. For example, concerning function, such life-sustaining machines as ventilators call for much more safety work than do electrocardiogram machines. Or a large machine may decrease the personnel's work space in an already tight patient unit, thereby impeding work efficiency and work flow. Storage may be a problem, so that equipment may be stored in an area not usually used—which creates delays in machine delivery. New machinery often requires extensive orientation of staff as to its safe use and the learning of new skills, and may necessitate the incorporation of personnel with different skills on the ward. More often than not, a period of time is required to work out the new division of labor, determine the machine's reliability, and so on. Where there are several types and models of a machine, staff must learn the idiosyncrasies of the different models and their appropriate software. For instance, in 1983, there were twenty-two different models of electronic intravenous infusion regulator pumps produced by fourteen different manufacturers (Huey, 1983). Machines placed permanently in the body (for example, a cardiac pacemaker) call for both machine safety and the patient's physical safety that extend beyond hospitalization, since kin and patient must be taught or "trained" to do the safety work at home. Then an organizational mechanism must also be developed so that the professionals can successfully monitor, prevent, and rectify risks when a patient with the pacemaker is at home.

As we have noted, medical machines are used after the models are first experimentally tried, then manufactured, sold, installed, operated, and monitored for their efficiency and safety. But then they must be serviced and repaired, as well as stored and kept supplied with parts. When newer models of machines are produced, the old ones are later traded or sold, and finally disposed of when too old or obsolete.

Just from the varieties of work involved in handling this machinery in the hospital itself, one can sense the great varieties of safety work required and engaged in by many persons and the large number of organizational arrangements—both inside and outside of hospitals—upon which this work rests. The work can be usefully discussed in terms of a threefold classification: (1) machine production safety, (2) machine-tending safety, and (3) machine-body-tending safety (Strauss, Fagerhaugh, Suczek, and Wiener, 1985).

Machine Production Safety. Machine production safety involves ensuring that when machines are being invented and experimentally tested, they will be made safe for both the patient

and the users of the machines. They must also perform efficiently. Installing a machine in the hospital also involves safety.
Machine production safety is concerned with safety during the
process of innovating, manufacturing, selling and purchasing,
installing, and preparing the proper environment (space, light-
ing, electrical wiring, and so on). This type of safety work involves complex relationships not only with hospital departments
and services but also with manufacturers and governmental
regulatory agencies. During the machine innovation process,
physicians, allied professionals, and specialized engineers attempt to perfect the machine for efficiency and safety. There
is an ongoing exchange between manufacturer representatives
and health professionals so that the machine can be improved.
This exchange is important because only through actual use of
a machine can most clinical inadequacies and clinical risks be
discovered. It is impossible to anticipate all of them outside of
the clinical setting.

Not infrequently, improvements are made by the users.
Some of these improvements get incorporated into the next
round of machine productions. For example, in the clinical situation, alarms for signaling the users of impending danger may
be insufficient in number, so that a bioengineer at the hospital
may devise and add new alarms. These improvements may be
adopted later by the manufacturer. Or, although a machine may
be proven safe in test situations and meet safety regulations,
unexpected contingencies may affect its efficiency. For example, the amount of insulation to protect the machine's functioning from outside electrical magnetic interference may be quite
adequate under test conditions but may prove very inadequate
when used in a hospital located near a television transmission
station.

When safety hazards are discovered, then a complex communication mechanism is required to cope with them. This must
be set up among producers, safety regulatory agencies, hospitals
and other users, as well as in conjunction with communications
within the hospital itself. This communication mechanism deals
with the specific hazards and how to rectify them; it also may
involve recalling a machine or its parts. Given the large numbers

of machines and related software, the safety communication mechanisms in hospitals are numerous. The great number of safety bulletins circulated in hospitals are witness to that.

Since most machinery is powered by electricity, safety work begins with proper electrical wiring and a back-up system for generating electricity to take over whenever a power blackout or shortage occurs. There are also requirements for the training and drilling of all hospital workers for emergency action, and for minimizing and preventing dangers should a power blackout occur. Our interviews and observations during and after a power failure at a large medical center revealed not only a great number of unanticipated difficulties because of a lack of organizational arrangements for the emergency but also many organizational shortcomings that pertained to everyday clinical safety demands. Moreover, the usual hospital organization of separating hospital services into medical care services and support services, and thereby providing electrical back-up only to essential medical services, highlighted the importance of a medical service–support service linkage. After this power failure, the hospital administrators decided to rethink essential medical care services and support services since these were so closely linked. Fortunately, no serious clinical hazards had surfaced, and everybody was relieved that the power failure had occurred during the day when resources were high. This was not the case of a more dangerous power failure at another hospital, which occurred during the night, when resources were fewer.

Considering the many different properties of machines that pertain to safety, the purchase of machinery necessitates consultation among many of the hospital personnel and the advice of various technical experts. Even when machines are proven safe in test situations, as well as through long usage, and have been produced by reputable manufacturers, there may be manufacturing defects: for instance, ground wires disconnected, cords broken, and plugs improperly installed. Safety considerations actually necessitate that engineers test and evaluate every newly purchased machine for defects even before its use.

Machine-Tending Safety. Machine-tending safety involves the monitoring and servicing of machines for their safety and efficiency, and keeping them supplied with parts, storing them, and later disposing of them when old and obsolete. Just as machine production safety calls for complex relationships among producers, hospitals, and repairers and suppliers within and outside the hospital, so does machine-tending safety. Whenever possible, hospital administration attempts to have in place institutionalized means for the selection, servicing, repairing, and monitoring of machinery. However, the development of adequate institutional arrangements to assure machine-tending safety is potentially fraught with difficulty. This is not only because of the great diversity in kinds and models of machinery produced by the considerable number of companies but also because of the rapid diffusion of these machines. In turn, this ever-changing diversity tends to produce a lag in organizational resources and institutional arrangements needed to cope with the safety tasks within hospitals, and within industry too.

For instance, an engineer was interviewed while he was installing an up-to-the-minute, latest computerized x-ray machine. A recent technological breakthrough had led to production and development of this particular model, which incorporated this technology. A race to be first between this company and another occurred. During the race, a handful of the best technicians were retrained to install and service the new machine in hospitals. Whenever one was installed, they were actually all there. At the time, four such machines had been installed throughout the country. When asked what would happen if a machine malfunction occurred, the team admitted there might be some delay since the number of trained technicians was still small and also, since the technology was so new, even well-trained radiology technicians ordinarily would not be able to remedy the problem. Asked about the interface of hospital personnel to their company, they replied that this was within the jurisdiction of the company's sales department, although they also said there was even some lag in updating the sales personnel on the new technology. Such a lag in knowledge and institutional arrangement between producers and health professional users is not uncommon.

Although hospital administrators attempt to maximize

safety by centralizing control over aspects of machine tending-
safety, that is not easy. Why? First, each medical specialty service tends to think its safety concerns are unique, a belief based
on experiential knowledge of working with a given type or model
of machine in relation to various illnesses. For example, in one
hospital at which we observed, efforts were made by the administrators to standardize cardiovascular monitors for all intensive care units, since it was reasoned this would assure better servicing and repairing. Consensus among the staff could
not, however, be reached because each ICU felt its clinical needs
were unique and could not be met by any single company's product. Since producers do compete for markets—which has the
consequence that models eventually improve—the staff did not
want to be saddled with one company's product should a safer
and more efficient model be obtainable from another company.
Also, each department had different machine priorities. Some,
for instance, had newer generations of cardiovascular monitors,
therefore preferred expending resources on the purchase of other
equipment.

There is a second condition impeding centralized control
of machines. Although many hospitals now employ safety engineers, bioengineers, and technicians to service and repair machines, those resources are rarely sufficient because new technology is constantly introduced to the wards. Its rapid absorption
is hastened in part by hospital personnel, especially the physicians, in their desire to have the "latest"—and presumably the
safest—in this fast-moving equipment market. Moreover, many
hospitals compete to attract both physicians and patients by having the newest equipment. At the same time, new technology
makes machinery rapidly obsolete, yet cost considerations may
prevent replacement of precisely those particular machines that
break down with frequency. Also, parts necessary to repair them
are not always available because of their relatively great age.
Even though hospital administrators may be well aware of the
necessity for expanding the hospital machine-tending service,
in pace with the expanding technology, cost considerations may
force a less-than-adequate service. Although hospitals are increasingly building into their equipment purchases various con-

tract provisions for service and repair, the reliability of servicing and repairing by the companies varies widely. Also, the
developmental stage of a given machine will affect the reliability
of its servicing. Given these conditions, different kinds of organizational arrangements have developed. Some are standardized, but ad hoc arrangements are usual. Informal systems
develop among various personnel, departments, and companies,
to cope with the inevitable shortcomings of more formal arrangements.

Storage of machine parts continually grows in complexity.
And the rapid occurrence of obsolete space in hospitals is amazing. For instance, six months after opening a new intensive care
unit, it may overflow with new supplies, while every nook and
cranny and the hallway itself will be cluttered with new or
standby machinery.

Then again, the supplying of machine parts and supplies
is extremely complicated, since the producing companies themselves depend on other companies for machine parts. So, hospital
wards turn toward multiple suppliers and make various kinds
of arrangements with them to meet their own needs. Supplies
can come from the hospital storehouses located outside the
hospital or from central supply in the hospital—as well as from
companies producing the machine, companies producing machine parts, hospital supply vendors, and machine rental companies. Each supply source may be affected by contingencies
that delay its delivery of supplies. The sources may have to
prepare its supplies, using machines that often break down. In
the central supply units, for example, the cleaning, packaging,
sterilizing, and delivery of supplies mostly depend on machinery.
(In one otherwise well-equipped hospital at which we observed,
this department was burdened with an obsolete sterilizer, inadequate for the volume of goods being sterilized. This necessitated making arrangements with other hospitals to cope with
the problem while awaiting the installation of a new sterilizer.)
Once supplies are delivered to a unit, a system of familiarizing
the staff as to their storage site is required, since locating supplies is extremely important on fast-moving hospital units where
speed of action is essential for safety.

The inadequacies of repair services and supply services require that the staff, particularly the nurses, remedy the shortcomings. Staff engage in preventing shortages of supplies and goods by hoarding ("squirreling"). Another common method of coping with shortage is by making informal arrangements with another department to borrow machines and parts. Not infrequently, tensions between departments and services occur when equipment is not quickly returned, gets lost, or is returned in defective condition. An enormous amount of time can be spent in remedying poor servicing. At one ICU where the problem was maximized by an unreliable repair service and old equipment, the charge nurse calculated that frequently she would spend two of every eight hours on problems related to machine maintenance. She would locate substitute machines for a malfunctioning one or even cannibalize another machine to create a functioning one.

Machine-Body-Tending Safety. Machine-body-tending safety involves the clinical applications of machines for diagnosis, monitoring, palliation, therapy, and the maintenance of life. This third type of work includes several subtypes of work that are particularly relevant to our discussion: setting up the machines and other necessary equipment and procedures; connecting and removing bodies to and from machines; informing patients about the machines and their own responsibilities in ensuring safety; calming patients' anxieties; monitoring both patients and the machines for clinical safety; assessing and monitoring the machine products (films, printouts, and so on); coordinating patients' schedules with the use of machines; attending to bodily discomfort while patients are on machines; and teaching patients and their kin how to use machinery if it is to be used at home. The staff (patients too) are largely and solely responsible for machine-body-tending safety. However, that work is closely linked with both machine production safety and machine-tending safety. Consequently, inadequacies in the latter two can adversely affect the former.

Moreover, machines are almost always used in conjunction with drugs and other medical procedures. This calls for an additionally complex task structure. In places like the ICU, machine-body-tending safety requires high skill and attention for assessing, monitoring, and rectifying possible risks and errors. Witness a Swan-Ganz catheter for monitoring the cardiovascular system, where some twelve possible risks can arise— either from connections of the equipment and machine or the patient-machine connection itself—for which there are some twenty-six causes and an equally long list of actions to rectify the causes (Hathaway, 1978). Or in the case of ventilators, there are some six machine-machine and machine-connection sites, which may be highly risky to the patient should they be accidentally disconnected (Janowski, 1984a).

Nurses, Technicians, Physicians, and Safety Work

The interaction of hazard sources places a heavy burden on the nursing staff. Nurses are on the front lines of the wards in spite of support services that can be utilized (technicians who repair and service the machinery, or the environmental safety engineers who help with other problems). They must, and of course if well trained and experienced do, have a level of technical understanding sufficient to identify both potential risks and their probable causes in order to utilize the technician more efficiently. Of particular significance to the interface of machine tending/machine-body tending is the burgeoning of new types of paraprofessionals and technicians. The latter include bioequipment technicians, special radiology technicians, heart catheterization laboratory technicians, and dialysis technicians. The training and language of these specialists are quite alien to that of most health professionals. Hence, misunderstanding and misexpectation by both sides in relation to safety work is not unusual (Holloway, 1979; Schreiber and others, 1981; Willens, 1982). In our interviews, the biomedical technicians stated that the most difficult aspect of their work was not only learning the nurses' limits of technical knowledge, although this varied widely from nurse to nurse, but also how to interact with all the health professionals and particularly the patients. The technicians and the bioengineers have similar problems with physicians, but not so much on a day-to-day basis. To add to their problems, the technicians usually worked with nurses under conditions where quick action was required and so nurses' patience was very low.

The assure the clinical safety for groups of patients is additionally difficult. Risk decisions may then become a heavy burden for staff members. Thus, in the ICU discussed earlier, the staff that was saddled with old machinery attempted to match resources with the hazard profiles of its patients. While a patient was in a high-risk state, he or she was cared for on a more efficient machine but once stabilized was shifted to an older and less efficient one. Risk decisions were difficult to make on this ward whenever a machine could not be matched with a hazard profile.

The sheer increase in the kinds of work necessary for maximizing clinical safety and the parallel complexity of hospital organization necessary for doing that have greatly altered medical/nursing work and patient care. In acute hospitals, nursing tasks for technology-related clinical tasks are constantly growing. (Some sectors of nursing have been alarmed by the increase in technology that is forcing nurses increasingly to become machine tenders. This is leading, it is asserted, to the neglect of patients' psychosocial needs and the dehumanizing of care; see Christman, 1978; Levine, M. E., 1980; Vecchio, 1977; Zemaitis, 1982.) Out of necessity, nurses also have become increasingly concerned with and skilled in carrying out coordination tasks, and such tasks as "product evaluation" (selecting the most safe, effective, and economical product). Although many nonnursing tasks (cleaning and getting supplies) are delegated more and more to nonnursing personnel, this has resulted in the nurses having to work through various levels of hospital personnel in order to obtain goods and services. This has resulted also in much frustration over the negotiations necessary for bringing about mandatory changes in work arrangements.

The pace of clinical tasks in the face of nursing shortages and the daily frustration of coping with complex organizations have caused many nurses to leave acute care nursing. As an alternative, they work in hospitals on a temporary basis, getting these jobs through employment agencies and registries.

More often than not, the temporary nurses hop from job to job within different hospitals. The growth in their numbers is partly because their use of employment agencies permits them more flexibility in social and life-style needs (Blackburn, 1980; Langford and Prescott, 1979; Prescott, 1979, 1982). Though efforts have been made by some agencies to assure the competencies of the temporary workers, their efforts are quite insufficient for meeting today's increasing requirements for clinical safety within the hospitals.

We have focused in the last pages especially on the safety work of nurses, since they carry out the bulk of the hourly and daily tasks of patient care. In passing, let us at least note and underline the safety work of physicians. Perhaps a contrast with yesteryear may help here. Lewis Thomas has described how sixty years ago physicians like his father were skilled at diagnosis but had virtually no effective therapeutic agents at their disposal. This situation had not changed even when he was a medical student—and did not change substantially until the 1950s. When Strauss studied medical students in the late 1950s (Becker, Geer, Hughes, and Strauss, 1961), he remembers the two major types of cautionary tales told by the faculty: diagnostic errors and terrible treatment errors that resulted in harm or death. Today the physicians are trained to acquaint themselves with the diagnostic and treatment hazards that characterize their (often specialized) practices. This entails avoiding procedural, technical, and pharmaceutical mismanagement, and thus involves appropriate and effective monitoring, assessing, managing of error, and rectifying of error. In short, they are engaging in the same basic work processes as the nurses, but, of course, their safety tasks are quite different in detail and organization. Physicians' perspectives, as well as their knowledge about diagnostic maneuvers and treatment modes, are necessarily somewhat different and often more extensive. However, sometimes in certain regards their skills are lesser, as with machine tending, machine-body work, or the utilization of machines. Yet, like the nurses, they, too, learn about medical equipment from experience rather than through formal training.

Summary

A major focus of health professionals in hospitals is upon clinical safety. This entails diagnosing, treating, and palliating patients who are afflicted with disease in ways that maximize safety and minimize harm. The assurance of clinical safety is an extremely difficult enterprise because of the diverse sources of hazard (the illness of the patient; the behavior of the patient; the various diagnostic, palliative, and therapeutic interventions applied; the personnel; the environment; and the institutional arrangements) as well as their complex interactions. Also, these hazards vary widely in their gravity, specificity, controllability, predictability, and rectifiability. All of this is taken into account in working out the clinical task structure. We suggested making this more explicit by the use of a "potential hazard profile" for each patient. To carry out the safety work involves the very complex coordination of bundles of tasks engaged in by the many workers. Besides these points, in this chapter we have discussed various types of safety work that are involved in using machines and the many contingencies attending the use of these machines that pose problems for giving safe patient care.

4

~~~~~~

Processes for Controlling Hazards

The guarantee of a successful trajectory for a serious illness requires an elaborate network composed of many kinds—and levels—of workers who are engaged in the safety work processes: assessing, preventing, monitoring, and rectifying the many interacting sources of hazard. In this chapter these work processes will be further examined, with particular emphasis on the interactional and organizational aspects of hospitals that impinge on them. We shall also discuss another feature of rendering trajectories less hazardous: the information work that is so much part and parcel of the work processes and of the staff's total activity.

Aside from preventing hazards, their accurate, efficient, and intelligent assessing and monitoring are the bedrock of clinical safety. Those two work processes reduce errors and the consequent problems of rectifying errors. Besides, if assessing and monitoring are deficient, then the legal and identity safety of the professionals, as well as their reputations and that of the particular workplaces, are endangered.

Distinction Between Assessing and Monitoring

Assessing and monitoring are interrelated processes, often occurring simultaneously. Hence those terms are frequently used synonymously. They are confused in usage by hospital personnel; perhaps this is because both activities require some criteria for safety limits and both involve the use of senses (eye, ear, touch, and smell) and measures that use various instrumentalities (procedures, techniques, medical devices). Although closely related, nevertheless the two are analytically distinct.

84

Assessing clinical hazards refers to both establishing the basic cause (or causes) of the illness that is endangering a patient and determining the appropriate treatment for managing the illness and its associated hazards. To this end, information is gathered through various instrumentalities. After analyzing and interpreting the information, judgments are made as to causes of the illness, and the gravity, controllability, and rectifiability of its dangers. Information is also gathered regarding available interventions and the possible risks associated with them. The appropriate interventions are judged by weighing and balancing their risks against dangers from the illness itself.

Judgments about causes of the illness and the associated danger priorities are, of course, based on knowledge about why dangers occur, as well as how they are manifested by the various bodily and emotional responses of the patient. Judgments are also based on information from various diagnostic measures. In addition, knowledge about what other dangers are likely to occur as this particular illness unfolds influences a judgment. Changes in body signs and symptoms, along with measures from various instrumentalities, are used to assess the progression of the illness and its related dangers, whether they are increasing or decreasing.

These assessments then establish priorities of hazards and the necessary actions to be taken by the many workers to control the dangers and risks within a manageable safety limit. In short, assessment implies a very high level of reasoning and cognition.

Monitoring is a more diffuse term, used in various contexts by hospital workers. Regardless of context, the term generally refers to some form of the following actions: observing, scanning, examining, checking, reviewing, recording, and overseeing and supervising of objects, persons, and events. Those actions more or less refer to the tracking of specific items and indicators associated with a potential hazard. Based on a prior assessment of anticipated danger and risk, certain items and indicators are then identified as important to track. This prior assessment determines the numbers of items and indicators to be tracked, how frequently, and for how long. Some are tracked very frequently because of their salience, others routinely. An interpretive process is involved, but the main emphasis is on tracking in order to prevent some potential danger or risk getting "out of hand." More often than not, the totality of tracked items and indicators is used when making a new assessment as to whether the dangers and risks are decreasing or increasing.

The activities involved in assessing and monitoring involve criteria of safety and interpretation. The activities also vary in level and scope. Moreover, effective and accurate assessment rests on effective and accurate monitoring—but the reverse is also true. Hence, a continual assessing and monitoring, reassessing and remonitoring ordinarily occur throughout the entire course of any illness. Of course, readjusting and rectifying often occur during the remonitoring and the reassessing.

Rectifying the Illness Trajectory

Rectifying refers to those actions that correct, readjust, and reregulate something that has gone wrong, or is going out of alignment, that may endanger the patient. Effective rectification of an endangered trajectory rests on an accurate assessment of its possible rectifiability—that is, the extent to which dangers associated with the illness can be corrected or reversed. This assessment involves the degree (complete-minimal), rate (rapid-slow), and duration (long-short) of correction or reversal of the endangered trajectory. Rectification efforts vary widely by disease and trajectory phases (whether early or late), as well as state of the art of the rectification measures that are utilized in reversing and controlling an endangered trajectory.

Thus, a number of variables pertaining to the degree, rate, and duration of rectifiability must be assessed. They include the following:

- The patient's hazard profile at the time of admission to the hospital.
- The reliability of various rectification measures and the extent to which they can rectify the assessed dangers.
- The risks (clinical, comfort, identity and biographical, legal and financial) associated with the rectification measures

themselves, as well as the extent to which they can be effectively controlled/corrected over the short- and long-term trajectory.

- The required resources and work organization in the rectification process available for the staff, patient, and family over both the short- and long-term trajectory.

These variables are taken into account in selecting the appropriate rectification interventions.

An important subprocess involved in rectifiability assessment is the weighing and balancing of these variables. It is also necessary to estimate how these variables interact in affecting the degree, rate, and duration of rectification. Staffs also estimate the risks associated with one or combinations of rectification measures, and what risks and/or aspects of rectifiability might be put in jeopardy in attempting to reverse and control an endangered trajectory. Because of today's life-extending and life-saving capabilities and the many rectification measures now available (all having some risks), certain moral and ethical issues have arisen. These pertain especially to the question of *appropriate rectifiability limits*. That term refers to whether rectification efforts should be continued, and for how long, given the perceived gravity of hazards associated with given rectification measures. The making of decisions about appropriate rectification limits is fraught with conflict, because definitions of appropriateness and risk balancing may vary widely among staff, patients, and families. Of course, these issues are also matters of bioethical, legislative, and judicial concern.

An orderly assessment involving all the variables is desirable. However, unexpected turns of the trajectory may prevent this because hazards have temporal rectification limits: reversing a hazard must occur within a given time before irreparable damage is done. When a danger is grave and becoming rapidly worse, the scope of rectifiability assessment is greatly restricted. For instance, in emergency rooms and intensive care units, patients are very often admitted in dire conditions, so there is little time to make extensive assessments. This is also true of delivery rooms where extensively damaged infants must be worked on speedily to be saved. In general, under conditions when unexpected hazards are rapidly increasing and when a patient is admitted to the hospital in a grave state—which is rapidly becoming worse—then the rectification focus is on lifesaving. In-depth rectification assessments occur only later.

Since effective rectification of an endangered trajectory depends on specialized resources, assessment of their availability and reliability is essential. This assessment is particularly important in assuring that intervention risks are efficiently managed. The state of the art of a given intervention is not the only factor here; cost considerations are also important. Thus, limitations of funding for health insurance and/or limitations imposed by governmental cost policies may reduce the intervention options. Aside from the usual resource problems for effective rectification of still-to-be-delineated risks that are associated with new technological interventions, some technologies call for material resources that are in short supply. A current, highly publicized example is the scarcity of organs for transplants.

Special problems attend the issue of assessing the reliability and the appropriateness of various rectifying interventions. The rapidity of new knowledge and the development of new rectifying measures constantly alter definitions of appropriateness— not to mention the controversies and debates among health professionals over this definitional issue. These controversies are widespread. For example, at the 1983 Scientific Session of the American Heart Association, held on May 12, 1983, the entire session was devoted to diagnostic and treatment controversies in cardiology. The following topics were debated in an attempt to delineate conditions under which given interventions are appropriate:

- "Echocardiography has made routine preoperative catheterization angiography unnecessary."
- "Pacemakers are grossly overutilized."
- "Echocardiography has made routine preoperative catheterization angiography unnecessary in congenital heart disease."

- "Risk factors can be modified to help prevent coronary heart disease."
- "Intracoronary streptokinase should be routinely used early in the course of myocardial infarcts."
- "There are drugs that can be used to salvage eschemic myocardium in man."
- "Unstable angina should be managed acutely with coronary graft surgery."
- "Coronary arteriography should be routinely performed in patients with clinical evidence of coronary artery disease."

That type of debate is also occurring in many of the other medical specialties.

Aside from purely medical and technical definitions of appropriateness, these definitions can have social dimensions that may be altered by changes in social conditions. For example, radical mastectomy was formerly the accepted intervention for cancer of the breast, but today a larger number of treatment options are offered, partly as a result of new knowledge and treatments but also because of both the consumer rights movement and the women's health advocacy groups.

Of growing importance in rectifiability assessment are the professionals' contributory assessments of patients' and families' capabilities, as well as resources (psychological, physical, medical, social, and economic), for carrying out necessary medical regimens during nonacute phases of the illnesses. Of special importance then is an evaluation of the appropriateness and effectiveness of patient-staff interactions as these pertain to teaching, reassuring, and supporting patients/families so that they more effectively carry out medical regimens. As mentioned earlier, many difficulties affect making such long-term rectifiability assessments. The further the illness extends, the more problematic becomes this assessment. When new technology is applied, there are many additional unknowns concerning the regimen. Even if the necessary skills and resources are known, health resources lying outside the hospital may not actually be brought into play when the ill are coping with regimen requirements at home (Corbin and Strauss, 1985; Lubkin, 1986).

Assessing Risk Consequences

An important and often difficult aspect of trajectory management is the assessing of risk consequences. Since many interventions carry with them potential risk consequences, assessment of these consequences involves weighing and balancing two or more of them, then making decisions about which interventions are actually to be risked. The consequences may be physical, such as a high probability of another illness developing that then may impact on the patient's identity, or cause undue financial burden, or precipitate legal or bioethical risks. In addition, since patient care is given within an organizational context, the personnel's own identity risks and estimates of risks to the organization of their work or their interactions also enter into their weighing and balancing of risks. The difficulties of risk assessment are due in part to the fact that different parties involved in the care (patients, family, doctors, nurses, social workers, technicians) all engage in the assessment but may actually be weighing different risks and different sets of consequences. Even when they weigh the same consequences of the same risk, they may weigh these quite differently. Conflicts can arise when each is not aware of the other's weighing, or its grounds.

The doctor may be weighing the medical risks of one type of medical intervention over another type purely on medical grounds or may be concerned with cost, but the patient may be weighing the risks as they affect his or her own identity. Generally, patients are assessing and balancing body discomfort against illness control, as well as the identity, composure, and staff-patient interactional risks, and making decisions about what is more important and what to risk. For instance, a patient may refuse a particularly discomforting or painful procedure, although aware that this might result in slowing the control of illness and even result in damaging interactions with the staff.

The latter are weighing some or all of these same items, but they sometimes weigh them differently than the patients.

They are also assessing and balancing risk consequences pertaining to their own identities and composure, as well as to staff-staff interactions. In addition, since they are responsible for groups of patients, decisions about risk have to be made about what aspect of a given patient's situation will be risked in favor of another's greater safety. For instance, should they risk damage to the identity and composure of one patient in order to better control another patient's illness? (This is another example of the implicit competition of patients for staff attention and resources.) The morale of the staff and composure of the total unit can be balanced against the continued presence of deteriorating patients, with even very conscientious staff eventually risking the composure and identity of these patients so as not to risk the morale and composure of the total staff. Finally, there is a legal risk that sometimes enters into this balancing by staff members.

To illustrate the various combinations of balancing that can be observed on wards, we have devised a risk-balancing matrix, as shown in Exhibit 2. If we place an X pertaining to how each person assesses these consequences, on a scale from high to low, then discrepancies among the various interactional parties can be identified. Here are a couple of instances: a patient chooses body comfort over smooth interaction with the staff, or over cost; the nurses emphasize minimizing a dying patient's discomfort while the physician may be emphasizing the "saving" of the patient. Identifying such differences on a balancing matrix might well prove useful to help resolve conflicts among the differently defining parties. The head nurse might take responsibility for the gathering of necessary information—to discover agreements and disagreements, and over which items. Once this information is assembled, it should be discussed openly, at a staff meeting if necessary, and a decision made about the most sensible source of action—including communicating this to the patient and family—in the light of the discussion. If this kind of procedure were properly institutionalized, it might improve the staff's sensitivity to potential disagreements concerning risk balancing, and so improve their clinical safety work.

Exhibit 2. Risk-Balancing Matrix.

Risk Consequences Regarding	Patient	Importance to			Others
		Family Members (1, 2, 3)	Doctors (1, 2, 3)	Nurses (1, 2, 3)	
High Patient's illness Low					
High Patient's behavior Low					
High Financial costs Low					
High Legal costs Low					
High Bioethical issues Low					
High Ward work Low					
High Other patients Low					
High Patient-staff interaction Low					
High Staff-staff interaction Low					

Clinical Risk Balancing

Purely on a clinical basis, the amount of balancing of clinical risk is immense. As noted previously, this is due to the complex interaction of multiple sources of hazards. Interventions made to control one bodily risk may create other risks to another body system. Thus, when many interventions are used, then the balancing of several risks requires intense assessing, preventing, monitoring, and rectifying. This is done to keep risks within a safe limit, so that no one risk gets out of balance.

Consider, for instance, two drugs that are commonly used for congestive heart failure, in which the heart is unable to pump an adequate supply of blood to meet the oxygen and nutritional needs of the body. These are digoxin, to improve heart action, and a diuretic, to assist the removal of pooled fluid in the body as a result of inadequate heart action. The cardiac drug, though extremely effective in improving heart action, has a potential for toxic reactions, such as changes in heart rhythm (potentially very dangerous), nausea, vomiting or diarrhea, visual disturbances, headache, lethargy, or mental confusion. The diuretic, though it aids in removing body fluid and sodium from the body, can cause potassium depletion and in addition may have harmful effects on kidney function. The diuretic drug also sensitizes the heart drug so that it has a greater potential for toxic reactions. Depletion of potassium can cause weakness, nausea, mental depression, and loss of appetite.

To keep the body in balance then calls for monitoring many items: the heart action (frequently with a cardiac monitor), urinary output, blood composition (reveals kidney function and electrolytes), and the patient's mental state and general bodily reactions. If diarrhea develops, then the patient must be closely monitored since the potassium loss can increase further through bowel action. In addition, the patient may be uncomfortable and weak from diarrhea, and is likely to have increased anxiety. A reassessment then has to be made. Decisions must be made about changing the drug or adding new ones, or additional testing may be necessary. Decisions are also made about the comfort work done both to relieve the patient's discomforts and increased anxiety. For all of that, these actions do not even include the safety work involved either in handling the oxygen device used for relieving respiratory distress or in using the cardiac monitoring machine.

Interactions of Safety Work Processes

The case just outlined illustrates the complicated interaction involved in the work of assessing, monitoring, preventing, and rectifying. Assessing determines the kinds and degrees of monitoring, preventing, and rectifying actions that need to be taken for controlling the assessed hazards. The monitoring work may require assessing, preventing, or rectifying. For instance, when a cardiac monitor is used, the other safety processes are involved so as to assure that the monitor is properly connected to the patient and is functioning accurately. The monitoring readouts are used to continually assess the patient's cardiac status. When this status is assessed as potentially dangerous, then different kinds of preventive, monitoring, and rectifying actions are called for. Interventions done to rectify a danger also require the other safety work processes. For instance, when using drugs or procedures, the reason for an intervention should be explained to reduce a patient's anxiety, discomforts associated with the procedure should be attended to, and the patient may need to be apprised of what kinds of bodily symptoms should be reported to the staff for minimizing a potentially untoward reaction. Finally, when monitoring, preventing, rectifying actions are taken, then their effectiveness or ineffectiveness must again be assessed. These assessments institute the cycle of work all over again.

This complex interaction occurs at both the overall trajectory and task levels. One can see the complexity of these work processes when a patient's overall bodily status is in a dangerous state. His or her anxiety is very high, and several interventions are rapidly and serially made. For instance, if someone who has congestive heart failure proves unexpectedly sensitive to a heart drug, then he or she may quickly develop a dangerous cardiac arrhythmia. Then the total safety process not only becomes speeded up but the entailed processes become much more complicated. Thus, a change in one process can affect other processes, and stress on the staff is increased.

Information Reliability: Problems and Issues

A considerable amount of information must be gathered in order to make accurate and effective assessments. The extent of information required, of course, varies widely by disease, and depends on whether the patient was admitted to the hospital with a definitive diagnosis or whether the diagnosis is still undetermined. In general, there is a routinized gathering of information, which is followed by a more focused gathering based on reasoning about probable causes.

The methods of gathering information involve a wide variety of instrumentalities. First of all, the assessors utilize their senses (eye, ear, touch, and smell) for symptoms and signs, often assisted by various instruments (such as stethoscope, otoscope) when examining the patient. Information is also gathered through an interview about past illness and social history. Other information is gathered through examining body products (urine, blood, body tissues) and through an array of machinery (like electrocardiography, radiography), procedures, and techniques. Reliability of information is crucial in making accurate assessments, yet there are many problems involved in establishing reliability.

There are many assessors who may vary greatly in their assessment capabilities. Hence, it may be necessary for someone to assess the reliability of the assessor's medical or nursing interview, observational skills, clinical knowledge, and sometimes even honesty or integrity. In general, health team members tend to accept each other's data as accurate on the assumption that each has had a common educational or clinical experience. More often than not, assessing and monitoring of another worker's (usually a peer's) reliability does not occur until some omission or error results in an unfavorable consequence, or some discrepancy is noted between another's observation and his or her own. Among nurses, this scrutiny tends to be more intensely focused on young graduate nurses, because their knowledge and skill may still be insufficient. However, newcomers on the ward are also watched for their general competence. In turn, the latter are also assessing the old-timers. In high-risk units, the newcomers all comment about the tensions related to "having to prove themselves." However, there is a general acceptance of reliability of assessments that rests also on the reluctance of professional groups to assess and monitor each other's performances (concerning physicians, see Freidson, 1976; Bosk, 1979). Although there are efforts to institute peer review of each other's performance, this is not easy to institute, because of the delicate peer interactions involved in these reviews. (This aspect will be more fully discussed in the next chapter.)

Indirectly, competence has been assessed through quality review mechanisms using the professional standard review. However, the reviews tend to be retrospective and focused on whether the care provided (including appropriateness of the assessment) met standards of accepted practice. Aside from being retrospective, the main focus has been on determining financial reimbursement for medical services rendered. At the peak of the relatively recent trend toward PSROs (Professional Standard Review Organizations), nurses were much involved in establishing standards of nursing care, including the appropriateness of assessment. And under the Diagnostic Related Group (DRG) approach, again, the major legislative focus is on issues of financial reimbursement, the difference being that standards now pertain to the kinds of diagnosis and treatment for different groups of illness that will be reimbursed. In addition, these reviews are prospective rather than retrospective. The relevant point here is that political and economic legislation can influence how assessments of hazards are managed, since cost considerations enter into the choice of kinds of information-gathering instrumentalities allowed.

Since patients also give information, their reliability as informants must be determined by the staff. Of course, under certain conditions accurate information may be difficult to attain, as when patients cannot speak or understand English, are hard-of-hearing, or are aphasic. Frequently, too, information is gathered under pressure of work, so it may be hurriedly gathered and though not necessarily inaccurate may be limited in depth.

It is interesting to note the frequency with which the phrase "the patient is a poor historian" is found written into hospital charts. Yet, our interviews with patients indicate that these were not at all poor historians. So, the bases for this misconception probably are the defective interviewing skills of interviewers or the time pressures emanating from staff work. Perhaps the generally tense interview situation itself may contribute to misconception, for most patients are interviewed shortly after their admissions to the hospital.

Other complicating reasons may affect the judgment made of patients as poor informants. Characteristically, many patients admitted to acute care hospitals have long histories of chronic illness. When interviewed, they have great difficulties in recalling all of their past treatments or drugs. Also, in order to get on with the business of living, they simply could not have afforded to focus constantly on their bodies and illnesses. Of far more far-reaching consequence for hospitalized care are the staff's negative judgments about patients being "hypochondriacs," "whiners," or "manipulators." The general tendency, then, will be for staff to discount or minimize a patient's expressed description of a hazard, although he or she may indeed be in grave danger.

It is important to recognize the information gathered from the various tests involves the skills of different professionals and often the use of various machines. Hence, the reliability of information depends upon the worker's performance and the correct functioning of the specific machine being utilized (such as its frequency of calibration). For instance, reliable information from diagnostic services rests on an adequate assessing and ultimately on the monitoring of both workers' performances and the diagnostic equipment. Then, of course, information from many diagnostic procedures involves interpretation by other expert assessors—radiologists, pathologists, and various technicians—so their interpretive reliability needs (ideally speaking) to be considered by those who act on their interpretations.

As noted in an earlier chapter, physicians may encounter difficulties when assessing the reliability of various diagnostic services and of the "expert" assessors, despite the guidelines and standards governing the operations of these services and the qualifications of their workers. Prior to an accreditation visit to such a service, there is usually a flurry of activity to improve its operations, but afterward the follow-up of monitoring of actual worker performance is likely to be somewhat lax. For instance, a supervisor at a cytology laboratory told us that her department had been accredited as meeting the guidelines and standards. On paper, all the cytology technicians were properly credentialed; yet she was burdened with two, of five, technicians whose performances were very poor. In spite of her careful work with them, their performances did not improve. Finally, she appealed to both the department head and the personnel for help, but this proved useless for solving the problem. In desperation, in order to prove her point, she thought of allowing the work done by these deficient workers to go through without the usual double- and triple-checking of it. However, her conscience would not allow her to use such tactics: a patient's life might be endangered, a wrong diagnosis would mean inappropriate treatments and unnecessary surgery. Here is an instance of reliability monitoring based on a personal sense of responsibility, but it was unsupported by an effectively organized, institutionalized mechanism. In general, then, doctors and nurses tend to accept at face value the diagnostic service reports. Inaccuracies are usually discovered when the information proves or seems discrepant with other information; then the test is repeated.

In sum, obtaining reliable information requires great diligence both by the information gatherer and the assessor of that information, since personal bias and the pressures of other work can affect its reliability. Also, the growing importance of information flowing in from the various diagnostic services does call for an increasingly organized accountability for assessing and monitoring the work organization, the worker performance, and the medical devices utilized in obtaining diagnostic information.

Complex Interaction of Safety Work
Processes and Its Consequences

The complex interaction of safety work processes, as discussed earlier, together with the growing numbers of hospitalized patients with highly unstable trajectories calls for the careful
monitoring of multiple items. These are monitored simultaneously by many personnel. Besides requiring a high degree of
discrimination, knowledge, and experience in order that accurate
assessments be made, this monitoring also depends on much
intra- and interteam communication.

The ICU flow sheet illustrates the growing complexity
of this monitoring. A flow sheet is a form used to keep track
of a variety of observations, measures, and interventions. Ten
years ago it was the size of an ordinary sheet of writing paper
attached to a clipboard, hung at the foot of the patient's bed.
Now its size is six to eight times larger and so requires a large
board, the width of the patient's bed. Observations and actions
taken by various staff members are recorded on this sizable sheet.

A central issue in the task structure that pertains to assessing and monitoring centers around the multitudes of items, persons, and events assessed and monitored throughout an illness
trajectory. All of this requires various types of workers (doctors, nurses, technicians, social workers) at various levels (staff
nurse, head nurse, intern, resident, attending physician). All
are involved in assessing, monitoring, and also rectifying the
various types of potential hazards, some of which are characterized by various interpretive complexities. At the same time, there
is much overlapping of responsibility for these safety tasks among
the different types and levels of workers.

For example, a staff nurse is engaged in assessing and
monitoring the cardiovascular system. She hooks the patient to
the cardiac monitor but checks out the machine first to see that
it is working properly. She connects the patient to the machine,
making sure that the connection leads are properly prepared
and placed on the patient's chest. She periodically scans the
monitor readout and checks the blood pressure and other bodily
reactions. She notes that the patient is becoming more anxious

and breathless. She checks the lung sounds and scans the monitor readouts. Based on these observations, she concludes that intervention is called for, but she cannot actually or legitimately do these interventions. So, the head nurse is consulted. The latter reviews the data and agrees with the staff nurse. The intern is called and reviews the nurse's observations, then makes his or her own observations. They discuss the problem together. The intern then decides that a resident physician should be consulted.

Each group and level of workers usually has boundaries placed on its safety limits, both in the scope and level of their work. These boundaries are determined by training, education, and legality. Because so many persons are involved in the safety tasks and because there are these safety boundaries, this situation usually necessitates that team members apprise each other. They also are supposed to seek assistance from appropriate groups and levels of groups whenever a safety limit exceeds their respective boundaries.

Because of the overlapping in this task structure, interactional difficulties can arise over such matters as (1) stepping beyond the respective safety boundaries, (2) not taking responsibility for assessing and monitoring hazards that lie within the boundary of a group, (3) forcing responsibilities on lower-level workers by a higher-level worker when they are believed to be beyond their scope and level, or (4) discounting the assessments made between different levels of workers. Indeed, intrastaff, and interstaff conflicts over the proper level and scope of respective boundaries are frequent.

A related condition is that experiential knowledge is very important to clinical competence and skill. Not infrequently some nurses may be more competent in assessing and monitoring certain types of danger than are the doctors. This situation is especially prevalent when the risks related to new technology are still being delineated by the ward's staff. Resentment by a physician can be high when a nurse—based on her experiential knowledge—makes suggestions for a more appropriate intervention or puts forth counterassessments. Resentment occurs here because the physician perceives or believes that the nurse has overstepped boundaries, but often the resentment seems to the nurse to be related to the physician's sense of status. This phenomenon is more apparent when the physicians are unfamiliar with the new technologies and new trajectories, and at the same time patients' hazard potentials are high. Young physicians are heard to mutter about some nurse engaging in "one-upmanship" or a "put-down." On the other hand, nurses resent that their assessments are ignored or not appreciated by physicians, or that one will accept a suggestion but with an accompanying sarcastic remark. Quite often such conflicts are discussed by nurses in terms of male dominance (Ashley, 1976; Cleland, 1981). Even when nurse-physician conflict at the unit level is minimal, the unequal experiential knowledge of a given nurse and a given doctor places a heavy burden on experienced nurses, for they must monitor the inexperienced physicians so as to prevent blunders. Thus, a frequently heard phrase in such wards as the ICU is "I get so tired of teaching interns."

This importance of experiential knowledge means that when first gaining experiential skills and knowledge, certain aspects of work may be neglected. Consequently, undue reliance will be placed on one method or another of assessing, monitoring, or rectifying. In machine-dense units, nurses comment that when gaining clinical competence, they first had to learn the intricacies of running the machines and of interpreting their readouts. At the time, they were preoccupied with what kinds of tracing indicate certain types of cardiac dysfunction, and what kinds of tracing can be attributed to artifacts, as well as what kinds of machine and machine-body connection failures can occur and how this is to be determined and corrected. Nurses admit to being so absorbed in "monitoring the monitor" at this point in their learning that their actual assessing and monitoring of patients was very limited. Later when they become competent and experienced, nurses and doctors can point to the "art" aspects of this work, adding (in their commentary) that machines must be seen in proper perspective—a tool among other tools (chiefly, the expert use of senses).

In short, a preoccupation with learning the intricacies of machine operation and of interpreting a machine's products may result in placing undue reliance on the machines, rather than taking into account other indicators of potential hazard. To illustrate: a new intern in an emergency room excitedly called for help in doing an immediate cardiac resuscitation, based on a cardiac monitor tracing. An experienced nurse, because of her observations of the patient, recognized that the monitor tracing was due to machine error. She yelled loudly to get the doctor's attention, "For God's sake! Will you look at the patient!" Or another, more catastrophic example: a cancerous tumor that had resulted in a greatly enlarged breast was dismissed as "nothing," despite repeated visits to a clinic by the unfortunate woman and repeated visual examinations by different physicians, because all placed complete reliance on her innocent-looking mammogram picture and interpretations of it. None of the physicians even did adequate breast examinations of the woman's fatally enlarged breast.

In spite of the overlapping of assessing and monitoring processes, each type of staff has major responsibilities for certain aspects of this safety work. The physician is mainly responsible for a patient's clinical safety, and certain types of technicians are responsible for machine and environmental safety. A notable difference in nurses' assessing and monitoring is that their work cuts across that of other groups, though patient comfort is usually understood to be mainly in their domain.

These differences in major responsibilities can result in the various types of personnel having different hazard priorities but without having any awareness of a patient's total trajectory. The personnel may also vary in their assessments of the danger/risk dimensions. In addition, they may vary in the importance that they attribute to indicators and measures of reliability and credibility. Thus, physicians tend to rely heavily on various laboratory tests for making assessments, whereas nurses are more likely to rely primarily on the patient's bodily and emotional responses. Therefore, different staff may ignore or miss a crucial assessment made by personnel from another specialist group. (Of course, patients too are making assessments, but these may not be accepted.) Interactional difficulties between staff members can arise from these differences. For example, a physician decides that a patient needs a potentially discomforting procedure, but the nurses believe its timing is inappropriate because the patient has been rendered sleepless and exhausted from previous invasive procedures, and that the patient's composure limit is near a breaking point.

The differences in work responsibilities may also result in different solutions. For example, nurses are largely responsible for preparing, hooking up, and monitoring the machines attached to patients. Thus risks arising from machine malfunctioning are often of greater concern to nurses than to doctors. In one situation that we observed, the nurses were tremendously concerned with potential dangers coming from several old cardiovascular monitors. These machines greatly increased the monitoring and rectifying work associated with them. While the physicians were sympathetic to the nurses, they were not sufficiently concerned to force the hospital administration to correct the situation. Such differences in judgment have consequences for the organization of safety work on the unit, for staff-staff interactions, and for the morale of the nursing staff.

Levels and Phases of Monitoring

The effectiveness of monitoring, of course, rests on the accuracy of an initial assessment concerning anticipated kinds of hazard. The monitoring is done for tracking the patient's bodily and psychological reactions to both the illness and the associated interventions, in order to provide a basis for determining the patient's overall current danger and risk status. Additionally, this monitoring is done to enhance alertness to potentially increased hazards.

Steps of the interpretative monitoring of hazards are usually phased in terms of (1) preventing, (2) might go wrong, (3) definitely going wrong, and (4) out of hand. Whenever possible, monitoring is directed at preventing anticipated dangers and risks from occurring. Not only are actions taken to prevent them, but items are monitored so that they remain within a given safety limit. Through the proper preventive actions and the simultaneous monitoring of danger and risk, the anticipated hazards can be held in check. Harking back to our discussion

of routine versus problematic trajectories: whenever the anticipated hazards of various trajectory phases can be mapped out
with explicit indicators and well-defined safety limits, then the
tracking of items can often be routinized.

Estimates are also made that something might be going
wrong. Are the monitored items at and remaining near the un-
safe side of a safety limit? Beyond what is the anticipated duration? Does a monitored item actually exceed the safety limit?
Is the patient developing a new, untoward reaction? If any of
those conditions exist, then a search follows to determine why.
Previously monitored items are reexamined for patterns of
change. New items may be examined, and further information
is sought by questioning and observing the patient. Judgments
are made concerning the corrective action to be taken within
the scope of the assessor's responsibilities, how long and intensely
the monitoring should continue, and when to report to another
level of health professional. If after the continued monitoring
there are indications that the situation has definitely gone wrong,
then the number of monitored items will increase; and assessments will be made as to the other levels or types of professionals
who must be consulted and notified, so that the danger or risk
can be contained.

In different diseases, a given hazard will vary in its speed
of traveling from "might go wrong" to "out of hand." For instance, for certain kinds of cardiac arrhythmias, precise, frequent monitoring and rapid interpretation in conjunction with
drug monitoring may be necessary. This is because of the various
kinds of potentially dangerous, rapidly appearing cardiac fibrilla-
tion and blocks. Thus, an initial assessment of controllability
must also include the conditions under which a given danger
can move rapidly from the danger phase to the next phase. Also
included in the original assessment is a need to anticipate the
kinds of resources necessary for maintaining the potential danger
within a given safety limit. When the corrective measures involve many personnel, then dallying over "might go wrong"
may result in insufficient time for organizing resources when
the patient actually enters the "definitely going wrong" stage.
On the other hand, some hazadous changes may occur more
slowly.

A definitive assessment of "in danger" may require several kinds of monitored items. The assessments may be highly ambiguous, bordering on the lower abnormal end of the normal-abnormal continuum. Also, of course, the patient's immediate bodily and psychological responses may not match the potential dangers as they would be in fact revealed by other measures and indicators, so that vigorous monitoring might comfortably be decreased. Or the danger progression is not readily discernible: for example, a very small hemorrhage that both the patient and staff may miss until the danger is well advanced.

In general, the nurses' monitoring tasks are mainly involved in the "preventing" and "might go wrong" phases. Also, as a given danger or risk moves from preventing, might go wrong, definitely going wrong, to out of hand, then a higher level of interpretative competence and skill is required. Our observations of difficulties between nurses and doctors suggest that most arise over differential assessments about the greater danger/risk phases. A nurse may assess that a given hazard that "might go wrong" is bordering on quickly becoming or is "definitely going wrong"—but may not be able to convince the physician. The nurse must call on her interactional skills to convince the physician, since legitimately to control the hazard does require the physician's cooperation. Nurses learn to cite a long list of signs and symptoms, and various laboratory and other measures to indicate the credibility of their judgments—but in a careful manner so that their interpretations are not misread as an intrusion on the physicians' diagnostic domain. As every nurse knows, night-shift nurses have a particularly difficult time convincing physicians that patients are in need of attention.

Types of Monitoring

In sum, the several kinds of monitoring tasks are varied and often difficult. There is the monitoring that is related to the patient's physical and psychological reactions to the disease and to the various clinical interventions. Since illness events are manifested often by some discomfort deriving from the disease itself, as well as those from the interventions, body comfort is likely to be of the utmost importance as an indicator. Besides, it is very important for patients themselves; indeed, they may have to tolerate much pain until they get well, so their comfort and composure limits must be constantly assessed, usually by the nurses. (Because comfort management is so important for nurses' work and for patients, a more detailed discussion of comfort work will be presented in Chapter Seven.)

Machine-related monitoring is very frequent in certain kinds of care units. Numerous monitoring tasks are related to machine functioning: monitoring for efficiency, accuracy, breakdown, and environmental factors which may compromise the equipment's functioning as well as endangering the patient and personnel; monitoring machine-body interfaces for proper connection; monitoring bodily reaction (pain and discomfort) to being connected to the machine; and monitoring psychological reactions to the machine. To assure safety, machines are produced with built-in safety monitors, such as flashing lights and buzzers to alert the monitoring agent that a machine is not functioning properly. However, these alarms can also malfunction so the machines may have to be set so as to monitor themselves, distinguishing true from false alarms.

Because patient care occurs in an organized work context wherein many levels and types of workers are working with different groups of patients, it is very important to monitor the hazard profiles in relation to available resources and required skills and competencies. Constant monitoring and reassessing are necessary to correctly match patients' changing profiles. Each staff member is monitoring and reassessing the implicit profiles of patients under his/her charge, while the head nurse is doing the same for all of them—and also for the unit as a whole. In addition, there is a monitoring of the general stress level, as it might affect the competence and the efficiency of the staff, as well as a monitoring of the staff's collective mood.

Since the task structure for assessing and monitoring often calls for the coordination of many workers and equipment, there must be a monitoring of the task structure itself. Moreover, there is a monitoring of all the necessary supplies and services, so that when hazards occur, they can be managed as efficiently as possible. To make matters more complex yet, there is finally the

monitoring of information. The amount of information transmission—in the form of verbal and written reports and recordings, machine printouts, laboratory reports, and so on—is enormous. The transmission is done both laterally and hierarchically.
It is engaged in by nurses, technicians, residents, attending physicians, pharmacists, bioengineers, and others. The transmission
of information is essential for both the short-term and long-term
management of trajectories. Omission or misinterpretation of
information, whether oral or written, can have dangerous and
even disastrous consequences for that management.

Staff Interaction in Rectification Work

Rectification work tends to provoke staff-staff interactional
strains, as well as personal and professional ones. Sometimes,
but not always, these are generated by having to rectify a hazard
stemming from an error made by someone. Then, blaming en-
sues, and ability and performances are brought into question.
(Error justification is discussed in Chapter Five.) For instance,
misassessment of a danger can delay prompt rectification and
further endanger a patient. Rectification—whether of an error
or not—also means taking action, and always there is the chance
of either having taken the wrong action or having misjudged
the risk consequences of a given action. The health worker then
must bear the burden of having misrectified.
Another feature of rectification work posing staff-staff difficulties is that often the assessing and monitoring may be done by
one type of worker, whereas the rectifying can really only be done
by another. Thus, a nurse may assess that a patient's discomfort
requires rectification and will apply interventions within her professional rectification limits but may judge that further rectification requires the use of drugs. This is a measure for which only
a physician can legally prescribe. Hence, when rectification involves having to convince another worker, of a higher level especially, that a danger or risk requires attention, then interactional difficulties are likely to arise. A physician may not agree
with a nurse's assessment or may delay action because of preoccupation with clinical problems of perceived higher priority.

Any number of things can go wrong in the task structure with regard to rectifying, just as with monitoring or assessing. The rectifier may not be readily available or may be unfamiliar with the particular danger. The task order may be out of line. The necessary supplies may have been forgotten. All of this calls for rectifying tasks—not to mention rectifying any new risks that may emerge. The latter include such interactional risks as lack of trust in the rectifier's ability or the wounding of identities by such sarcastic comments as, "Don't you know better?"

When clinical risks are involved, the emphasis tends to be on biophysical and technical medical/nursing tasks. Yet, most task structures also include safety tasks related to patients' biographical profiles and identity, to their bodily comfort, and to the composure of both the patients and staff. The same point also holds for rectification work: although biophysical risk has first priority in rectifying, other safety tasks are also very important. Quite often a patient is aware that something is going or has gone wrong, and needs rectification—but may not be rectified—so his or her anxiety is high. The staff's anxiety may also be high. All of this requires that the patient be reassured and that the staff be calm and composed; otherwise the organization of rectification work can become disrupted. Effective rectification calls for a high degree of psychosocial work by both the patient and the staff.

Rectifying the Task Structure: A Political Process

Effective rectification work may require an alteration of an existing task structure. This may involve realigning or changing some aspects of that structure—changing the various workers' responsibilities; changing how tasks are arranged among them, and how and what team members communicate about the risk aspects of work; changing, too, the materials or equipment used in the work, or the numbers and level of workers involved in given tasks. All of this means that someone needs to convince others that something requires changing in order to assure a genuinely effective task structure.

To bring about these necessary alterations may involve negotiations, not only among the health workers directly involved in a task but also among hospital administrators or middle managers from the various hospital services. Because of the complexity of many a task structure—which very frequently calls for aligning the work of many kinds and levels of workers—its rectification is inevitably a highly political process. Negotiations (bargaining, wheeling and dealing, compromising, making deals, making arrangements, mediating, power brokering, trading off, exchanging and engaging in collusion) usually are involved—both upward and downward—among the hospital's personnel. The greater the levels and kinds of workers involved in a task structure, the more complex becomes the negotiation around rectification. There will be greater variation not only in definitions of dangers and risks but also in how various persons choose to balance the risks.

Rectification of a clinical risk may also require that changes be made by the manufacturer of a given technology. The changes may require altering it for greater safety or altering the assessing, monitoring, and rectifying work done during the production itself, so that a safer product is assured. At a regulatory level, safety regulations may need to be added, deleted, or changed. This rectification of clinical hazards also requires that some representative of the hospital negotiates with producers and regulatory agencies. However, the process of negotiation begins at the ward level. Understandably, all of this is a highly political matter.

Information Work in Controlling Danger and Risks

The successful, safe management of illness also depends upon an effective flow of information among workers, patients, and their kin. The very fact that ''lack of communication'' or ''goof-ups in communication'' are frequently cited by workers when work goes awry and safety is imperiled indicates the importance of effective information. As noted by E. Gerson (1981), every kind of work involves production/consumption/use of information; hence the handling of information is part of the task structure of every kind of work.

The work of managing information has particular significance in the hospital's work because the safety work processes require immense amounts of accurate information. "Goof-ups" in information work can result in dire consequences to the patients, workers, and the hospital itself.

Trajectory management includes innumerable types of work with information: gathering, recording and assembling, acting on, transmitting to others, discussing, debating, reviewing, retrieving, and storing it. Moreover, there are several major kinds of information. There is first the vast amount of clinical/technical information pertaining to safe diagnosis and treatment work. A second kind of information is related to working with the behavior of the patient—that is, biographical and other information related to body comfort and psychological work. Third, there is information about organizational contingencies that affect work. And fourth, there is the combination of all these kinds of information, as they relate to task structures involved in doing the overall trajectory of work.

Every worker, including the patient, engages in information work, but each differs in the kinds engaged in. The division of labor pertaining to the work is determined in part by the worker's major responsibilities in the trajectory management but also is based on how his or her jobs overlap with that of others. Certain hospital personnel, such as those in the records department, are primarily concerned with reviewing patients' charts for certain types of information and with storing and retrieving information. Hospital administrators are concerned with receiving certain kinds of information, such as those related to allocation of resources, environmental safety, or legal and accreditation safety. Some workers are pivotal in giving or receiving information, especially the head nurses on patient care units, because they must process and coordinate information coming from many kinds of hospital departments and personnel.

Inherent structural conditions related to medical work and hospital organization can readily disrupt information flow and so affect the clinical safety of patients. The complexity of organization, with its many specialized workers and departments, requires the input and coordination of information from many kinds and levels of workers, but the workers are spread out spatially. This results in information flowing through a series of intermediary steps. Hence, opportunities for clarification of information are made difficult. Trajectory management in hospitals is done around the clock, seven days a week, but workers usually work eight-hour shifts and forty-hour weeks, and the schedules of some workers, such as physicians, may be highly variable. Flow of information may be disrupted during changes of shifts. Gaps in information can result because of workers' days off. Temporary workers who are filling in can readily disrupt information flow due to their unfamiliarity with the work processes. (As noted earlier, the contemporary trend toward hiring temporary nurses from commercial registries results in employing relatively untrained personnel even on wards where up-to-date, highly specific knowledge and information is requisite for full clinical safety.) Unavailability of a worker or the worker's being elsewhere are also common sources of information disruption. In short, the flow of information— to whom, by whom, where, and how—can be quite complex and must be taught and learned.

Task Structure and Information. At the task level, information work can consist of microtasks, although these differ somewhat by trajectory phases and miniphases. For instance, in diagnostic phases, the focal emphasis is on gathering information from various types of workers and then assembling and analyzing it. Minitasks are carried out both by patients and staff in gathering, assembling, and analyzing other information. Staff, of course, must be mindful of minitasks in their data-gathering encounters with patients; otherwise problems may arise when attempting to gather accurate information.

Analyzing the information for arriving at a course of action may require many informational tasks, including those involved in discussion and debates. Deciding on a course of action may require persuading, teaching, and negotiating with colleagues, patients, and kin. Once a course of action is taken, there will be informational work that relates to the treatment process, and to the monitoring and the evaluating of treatments. When the trajectory is routine, then information work can be highly standardized. However, when the trajectory is unfamiliar or the trajectory goes off course, then information work greatly increases.

Since tasks are part of a larger chain of work, any procedural work calls for different mixes of information/communication work done before, during, and after each task. Most tasks call for resources of space, personnel, equipment, and time. Sometimes workers must communicate either with members of other departmets or with workers in other echelons. Communication must take place between staff and patients as well as their kin—information must be shared and questions answered. Also, depending upon the nature of the work, information may be sought or offered: information about the safety of the equipment, or about a patient's physical or emotional states that might compromise or render the work risky. While carrying out the tasks, information is given to patients concerning what to anticipate and what actions they themselves must perform—"move your head," "hold your breath." When two or more workers are involved, there is communication about anticipated next steps and directions to others about performing certain minitasks. After the task is completed, there is further communication. There may be evaluative talks about the task performance, the result of the task, the further information that needs to be gathered, the anticipated next steps, and the information that must be monitored. When snags in the work are encountered, there may be sharp reprimands of "don't let it happen again" or communications about the work or the organizational rearrangements necessary to avoid snags and, of course, to maximize clinical safety.

Writing, Reading, and Talking: The Patient's Chart. The patient's medical record, or chart, is a pivotal instrument of information work. Since it is the official document and a major repository of information about the patient's hospitalization and since charts are filed at the nursing station on the ward, these charts and the nursing station itself are at the hub of the information work. Staff write in the charts, read them, review them, talk about information in them, and use them as a major tool in teaching. Further, since the charts are official documents, they are used as evidence in lawsuits; therefore, legal considerations influence what information is recorded in them. In addition, charts are used as evalutive tools in medical care. For instance, they are reviewed as part of quality control and are further reviewed by hospital accreditation agencies, such as the Joint Commission for Accrediting Hospitals. So the charts reveal much about what is regarded as accountable and nonaccountable information.

The charts, of course, contain information gathered by many workers. A physician will gather information pertaining to the patient's medical history and physical findings, possible diagnosis, courses of treatment, progress notes of patient's reactions to the illness and therapy, and any other associated physician's directives to others for carrying out courses of action (doctor's orders). A nurse's information includes observations of the patient's physical and emotional states, biographical information, nursing and medical tasks carried out, and the patient's response to these. Diagnostic test results are also included. Results of major treatment such as surgery are written up. Consultant's findings and recommendations are found there. Patient consent forms, signed by patients, for specific types of diagnostic tests or treatment are included. So is demographic information (age, sex, religion, and so on) and what kinds of insurance coverage the patients have.

Some kinds of information are written in standardized forms, though other kinds are written in familiar narrative form. There are also many types of flow sheets, in which prescribed kinds of information are recorded over a period of time, in order to provide a quick summary of patients' illness status and responses to therapy. The flow sheets are tailor-made for certain kinds of diseases, types of treatment, or levels of illness acuity, where specific types of information are crucial. In sum, these prescribed, standardized forms make accountability more likely and are designed ultimately to make the medical-nursing work more efficient and effective—and clinically safer.

The bulk of information, written and oral, pertains to

technical matters. Information about psychological work is usually transmitted orally to others, partly because much of it is implicit. Biographical information also, unless clearly relevant to
clinical care, is not written down but is transmitted orally.
Negative assessments of patients as persons, sometimes based
on moral judgments, tend to be transmitted orally as well. Frequently, however, they appear in charts in the form of complaints about patients being "difficult." Noticeably missing is
information about snags or botch-ups in the carrying out of
tasks, even when safety was involved. To take a simple case:
a physician may cause tissue damage and pain to the patient
while making a needle puncture to start an intravenous infusion. This information is often unrecorded, although the start-
ing of the intravenous infusion and the kind of solutions and
drugs added will be duly recorded. A nurse may comment verbally about this to others and thereafter monitor the needle site.
That the physician's job was incompetent can be gleaned from
a later recording made by the nurse, which notes that the area
around the puncture site is black-and-blue and indicates the kind
of action taken to rectify this condition.

On a fast-moving care unit it is often difficult to find time
to carefully read the charts. Yet given the truly vast amount
of information in many charts, an important aspect of information work is how to read and scan them in order to glean
significant information for organizing work. Of course, learning to efficiently read charts is based on being able to anticipate
what information is significant for organizing the given tasks.
More often than not, the significant information is transmitted
orally.

This great amount of information must be processed and
operationalized into action. It must be summarized as related
to work that must be done, noting how frequently and when
it is to be done. Doctors' orders are put into action by writing
out requests for equipment, resources, and drugs. Usually the
information is transcribed into a centralized form containing
pertinent information about the patient, the current and impending treatments, and the specific kinds of information that
must be monitored. This provides a quick summary for all

workers. However, those responsible for given patients are notified verbally about the upcoming work. Usually these latter kinds of informational work are done or supervised by the head nurse.

As to who reads whose recordings: nurses tend to be attentive to doctors' narrative notes, though doctors rarely read those of nurses. Physicians read those written by other physicians, paying particular attention to diagnostic reports. Nurses' recordings as done on flow sheets are usually read by physicians, too. Nurses read doctors' narrative reports, doctors' reports, and diagnostic results, since these are important guides in anticipating further information that they must gather and monitor. Further, nurses are responsible for operationalizing the information into tasks. In short, information is attended to only if directly related to major work responsibilities.

Organizational and Interactional Information. Since all of this work occurs within organizational and interactional contexts, the personnel require much information about both organizational functioning and their co-workers, such as work schedules of various departments and wards; or workers' competencies, incompetencies, and idiosyncracies. Some of this information is formally transmitted; however, much is informally learned and passed on. One can overhear physicians informing each other that a nurse on such-and-such unit is competent or incompetent, or is reliable, and how certain kinds of work are handled differently on different units. In their turn, nurses pass along similar information about physicians to other nurses. Moreover, personal information about individual physicians is learned as it is passed along: "he is a very formal person so you can't kid around." Workers pass along information about strategies that work and don't work, what can be negotiated and what can't. To give and receive all of this information is necessary for clinical tasks, since that determines the degree of explicitness required when giving directions, or indicating the necessary frequency of monitoring another person's work, or discussing someone's competency or reliability, and so forth. Such information is also important in reducing interactional tensions and conflicts, and for maintaining sentimental order on the wards.

Recording and Its Legal Consequences. Since patient's records
are used as evidence in lawsuits, there is a growing concern about
staff's work errors appearing in the actual recording, and so personnel or the hospital itself being found legally liable for these
errors. To protect themselves, workers must learn how to record,
what to record, and when to record. Increasingly, there are continuing education courses and seminars that address issues of
legal protection and documentation: how to avoid documentation errors and ambigous statements, how to improve clarity
and conciseness, and how to avoid risk of liability through errors of documentation. The great concern for legal liability in
recording is exemplified by an advertisement for a documentation seminar designed for nurses. The advertisement opens with
this statement: "Five of the scariest words in the English language are 'I'll see you in court.'" Nurse administrators and
supervisors are now consulting attorneys in order to avoid the
legal consequences of errors. One nursing supervisor stated in
dismay that there was a growing (legal liability) paranoia about
record keeping.

The importance of communication work can be found in
litigations where workers were found liable because of failures
in communication (Cushing, 1982). Although ultimately the
liabilities were based on faulty judgments, the errors involved
some communication errors. They include (1) omission of documentation (Groff, 1985); (2) failure to transmit information to
the proper person when time is of the essence; (3) failure to
transmit information regardless of contingencies that might have
presented barriers (such as a failure to locate the person who
is supposed to receive the message); (4) failure to properly assess
and listen to communication given by the patient, thereby delaying appropriate action; and (5) failure to read and note significant written information (the history), which resulted in the
delayed preventive measures. In essence, these errors are related
to gathering, reading, processing, and transmitting information.
The significant point here is that the work of communicating
is crucially linked to safety and to error management.

Patient/Staff Information Work. Throughout our chapters,
we have touched on minitasks concerning patient/staff infor-

mation. We have also discussed various trajectory phases when such information work was highly significant. For instance, that information can be important when difficult decisions must be made about diagnostic and treatment options, and when risk consequences must be disclosed. However, there is also the giving of information to assist patients in following the medical regimen just before their discharge from the hospital. This informational work is growing in importance with the increase in chronic illness; the work is usually categorized as "patient teaching." It entails gathering information about what the patient knows about the illness and its management, as well as making decisions about the appropriateness of kinds of information needed by the patient, the appropriateness of methods and approaches of transmitting this information, and the pacing in passing on information. "A patient's right to know the truth" not only hinges on such communication work but also relates to moral-ethical concerns regarding withholding information from patients, distorting information, and outright deception. If the work of passing information to patients before they leave the hospital is done poorly, or not at all, then the later risks and dangers to patients are enhanced.

A Few Last Questions Concerning Information Work. A focus on information work raises questions about many facets of this work. For instance, why are certain kinds of information work more important to some workers than others? Why do certain workers emphasize communication? For instance, nurses tend to be especially aware of it, because they function in a particularly important integrator and coordinator role, processing and transmitting information from and to many workers. They are also largely responsible for the caring work. Hence their training emphasizes communicating well in order to establish humanistic relationships and therapeutic communication with patients.

But to continue with the questions: What conditions prevail for accountable or nonaccountable information work? What are the consequences of doing or not doing certain kinds of information work? How are standardized information records developed, who reviews them and evaluates them? Why are they changed? How is information work learned, and taught, to whom, and by whom? How is it monitored and evaluated? Such questions are surely close to the heart of understanding the clinical safety issues in contemporary hospitals.

Summary

The formidable task of controlling the interrelated sources of hazards was examined by analyzing the major safety work processes—assessing, preventing, monitoring, and rectifying—and their crucial linkage to information work. How the safety work processes are interrelated, their linkage to information, and the various types and levels of work were discussed.

The discussion illustrated the uncertainties surrounding illnesses and technological interventions, the multiple kinds of risk consequences associated with the interventions, the organizational and interactional context in which hazards must be controlled, the wide variety of definitions of safety limits, and what can be risked among and between health professionals and patients. These concerns are taken into account in the risk balancing matrix to sensitize the staff to potential disgreements on definitions of risk and risk balancing, and to improve clinical safety and staff and patient interactions.

The interacting safety work processes result in much overlapping of work among staff, and between staff and patients. Therefore the improvement of hazard control requires that the division of labor be constantly negotiated and renegotiated among the involved parties.

Finally, information work was analyzed: its task structure, its variety and types, and the many contingencies that affect it.

5

∽∽∽∽∽∽∽∽∽∽∽∽∽∽∽∽∽∽∽∽∽∽∽∽∽

Preventing, Assessing, Monitoring, and Correcting Errors

In any occupation or organization the prevention and control of errors made by workers are important for maximizing safety. Particular occupations and organizations vary widely in the specific consequences that mistakes have for them, their workers, and their clients. In acute care hospitals today, the concern for errors made by personnel looms large because of two parallel developments. First, as we have amply seen, the expansion of technology increases potential hazards for the patients. Second, since our country is becoming increasingly litigious, there is a growing reliance on the judicial system for adjudicating perceived wrongs (mistakes of judgment or procedure) and injustices, and the consumer rights movement has hastened a greater awareness and less passive acceptance of medical errors. These developments have profoundly affected health care institutions and health care personnel as they struggle to prevent and manage error.

Legal Issues and Error

Since errors are involved in issues pertaining to cost, legality, moral-ethical matters, professional careers, and institutional reputations, the interaction of these safety concerns has created new risk concerns. For example, the fear of being found legally negligent because of error has forced hospital administrators and health workers to be more accountable in preventing errors through rules and regulations. These pertain to the skills and knowledge of personnel, their monitoring procedures, rectifying procedures, and so on, all of which are relevant to assuring safety. However, in order to assure legal protection against negligence attributed to error, the cost of health care has increased, because of higher liability insurance costs for hospitals and their health workers. Furthermore, the practice of "defensive" medicine may expose patients to increased numbers of diagnostic and monitoring tests, thereby not only increasing costs but exposing them to further potential hazards that are associated with medical technologies.

In consequence, over the last decades a growing emphasis has been placed by hospital administrators and personnel on the legal consequences of errors. An examination of journals published for hospital administrators, doctors, nurses, and the various technicians shows a steady increase in the number of articles addressed to the legal consequences of errors. These articles pertain to the kinds of and grounds for errors that constitute legal negligence, to the health team members held liable, and to the protective measures for assuring legal safety. Most health professional journals regularly feature by-line columns such as "Legally Speaking" or "Legal Side," which discuss legal cases involving various kinds of legally liable errors. Physicians are bitterly complaining about the "impossibly" high costs of their malpractice insurance. In nursing, there is a steady rise in the number of continuing education courses and conferences addressing various legal aspects of nursing practice. Nurses who have law degrees are also increasing in number.

These trends seem to point to medical and nursing errors as being legally defined rather than simply clinical, humanistic, or philosophical concerns. Not unlike the trends toward litigation that are affecting many other aspects of American life, the tendency to settle many aspects of health care on legal grounds has been very greatly extended. For example, legalism has strongly influenced decisions on moral/ethical issues of health care (Ladd, 1979). It is interesting to note that our own search through the medical and nursing literature that bears on mistakes and errors turned up relatively few articles and studies indexed under errors or mistakes; in contrast, a great range of types of errors were indexed under legal negligence and liability.

Because the consequences of errors are potentially fateful both for the patients and for the personnel making the errors, training of the latter emphasizes the skills and knowledge needed to prevent and minimize the probabilities of mistakes at work. In training, the consequences of error are underscored and often accompanied by horror stories used as "moral parables" (compare Bosk, 1979). This teaching emphasizes the professional and moral responsibilities for proper skills, knowledge, conscientiousness, and so on, in order to prevent errors. Given the current health scene, a more apt term for these teachings might be *legal liability parables.*

In short, sectors of medicine and nursing are seriously grappling with complexities involved in the legal practice of medicine and nursing, and the attendant moral-ethical issues. This is further attested by the existence of journals such as *The Journal of Medicine and Philosophy* and *Nursing Law and Ethics,* policy centers such as the Hastings Center, and the development of departments of bioethics at large medical centers. Although in the following discussion the legal aspects of error will not be our major focus, nevertheless since legalism is a strong force affecting error management, it and associated ethical issues must ultimately be taken into account in understanding the management of clinical errors.

Error Work

A central, inevitable activity of trajectory management is the management of clinical errors, or in our terminology *error work*. Errors are, of course, concerned with mistakes made by humans—something done wrong; either acts of omission or errors of judgment (misidentification, misinterpretation, and misconception). These may create or increase hazards to a patient, the staff, or the environment. Error work goes hand in hand with assessing, monitoring, and rectifying dangers and risks throughout the various trajectory phases. Understandably, this error work can constitute an onerous responsibility for staff.

Recollect that the work of assessing, monitoring, and rectifying hazards is based on the usual criteria of safety limits: the what, when, and why of something being safe or not safe; also what, why, when, where, and how the right and wrong way of doing something may cause or increase a hazard. Involved in error work, however, are normative criteria for making safety judgments and actions. A deviation from these normative criteria then constitutes error—consequently, something or someone will be held culpable for the error.

Therefore, the effective preventing, assessing, monitoring, and rectifying of errors are each directly related to how well hazards can be anticipated and mapped out throughout all the trajectory phases. Each is also directly related to how well these work processes are organized into a safe task structure. Then when errors do occur, they can be managed so that harm is held within rectifiably safe limits.

A paradoxical feature of effective error work is that it actually rests on the occurrence of past errors. This is because even though many hazards are anticipated and controlled in the experimental or developmental phases of new technology, unexpected errors inevitably occur when it is actually used with patients. Every new technology, of course, goes through a "working out of the bugs," or a trial and error phase, at which time various errors (hopefully, not serious) are made and then discovered. These can be of a technical-clinical nature or related to the given task structure and/or the organizational arrangements. Even with an old technology, new models or new parts (like connectors) are constantly being produced, so a period of trial and error for them is necessary. It is interesting to note that in the trial phase, personnel tend to define errors with some degree of leniency. Likewise, during this time patients and their families also tolerate errors with an amazing degree of stoicism and resignation.

The analytic point here is that definitions of error and culpability must be understood in their temporal contexts, and these definitions do change over time. They are tied directly to the developmental and usage phases of a given technology. Since both new or old technologies are used in many places under different sets of conditions, new and unexpected hazards are constantly being discovered. Thereafter, the discoveries are disseminated through the professional clinical journals, as well as through special journals and newsletters, such as *Professional Liability Newsletter, The Citation, Drug Alert, Devices and Techniques,* and through bulletins produced by such governmental agencies as the Food and Drug Administration. Effective error management, then, rests not only on communicating about errors within specified workplaces but also on effective communicating about past errors made in workplaces throughout the entire country. Nevertheless, given the rapid changes in technologies, keeping up-to-date on their possible errors represents a major problem for health personnel.

In general, after using technologies with patients who suffer from different illnesses, the various safety criteria—danger-safety limits, as well as necessary skills, knowledge, experience, and the organization of tasks to prevent, assess, monitor, and rectify hazards—are all established and become standard operative procedure. At this point in the technological process, certain acts and judgments made by workers are judged as error, and persons can therefore be reasonably judged as culpable.

The difficulty in doing effective error work, of course, is greatly increased by the predominance of acutely ill patients in the late phases of their chronic illnesses—often subject to uncontrolled and unexpected contingencies—and by the complex task structure of clinical safety work itself. Together these sources contribute to the difficulty of anticipating possible errors and actually rectifying them once they occur.

Disconnections of Ventilators: An Example of Complex Error Work

However much error may be of concern to health workers, they face inherent problems because of all the complexities of clinical care discussed earlier. An instructive illustration is provided by a study of accidental disconnection of the ventilators used in anesthesia and intensive care units. The study was made for the Food and Drug Administration by A. D. Little, Inc. (Cooper and Covialon, 1983).

Because ventilators are machines for saving and sustaining lives, disconnections of the machine-machine interface as well as patient-machine interface (there are ten vulnerable disconnections) can have fatal consequences. Of course, the most risky potential disconnection is the tracheal-machine connection for which an incision is made directly into the throat. In spite of the potentially fatal consequences of such disconnections, this study found that disconnections are considered minor events. They are rarely recorded in incident reports, unless an injury is serious and made as a result of either gross error or machine failure. Disconnections are such a common occurrence in intensive care units as to be considered routine. Most were found to be the tracheal-machine disconnections.

In order to prevent damage to patients, there are alarms to apprise workers of disconnections. Other methods of preventing errors include making the connection tight, as well as frequent monitoring of machine connections and of patient-machine connections. However, in this management of clinical safety, disconnections are not the only risk of concern. There are also risks related to the pain and discomfort of the patient, the other treatments and procedures involved in and around the tracheal-machine connections, and the infection control of the tracheal site as well as of the respiratory system. And, as always, there is also the issue of monetary cost. Thus, potential disconnections must be balanced against other risk concerns.

The researchers report that most disconnections were discovered via the alarms, yet most fatalities occurred while an alarm was turned off. The alarm was off because the clinicians would forget to turn it on after deactivating it when doing procedures such as suctioning or bagging or intubations. Often an alarm was turned off because of the frequency of false alarms, which had not only raised the noise level but unnecessarily alarmed the patients. Moreover, alarms on other ICU equipment, which also gave off numerous false alarms, had resulted in lessened sensitivity to alarms in general and therefore had delayed responsiveness to emergencies.

Although a tight tracheal-machine connection is desirable for preventing disconnections from occurring, most clinicians preferred a looser connection. This allowed for easy disconnection—in order to have access to the patient's airway to enable the necessary suctioning for keeping the airway open—as well as permitting other kinds of procedures. Moreover, a loose connection would prevent an extubation (expelling the tracheotomy tube) should the intrapulmonary pressure increase because of the patient's coughing or movement, tension in the tubing, or water having collected in the circuit. An extubation is considered more immediately serious than a disconnection. In addition, increased pressure can be very uncomfortable for the patient.

To prevent infections from a contaminated respiratory machine system, its parts are changed at frequent intervals, when sterile disposable parts are substituted. Because of cost considerations, these disposable parts may be resterilized and reused, but reused parts unfortunately tend to have loose connections. However, some clinicians believe the disposable components are inferior and result in ill-fitting connections, whether new or reused.

Manufacturers have attempted to remedy such potential disconnections. The study found that most personnel believed that reliance on alarms can create a false sense of security, which cannot replace close monitoring of machine functions and machine connections or of the patient. Some manufacturers have introduced antidisconnecting mechanisms (straps, hooks, adaptor knobs, elastic bands, spring and lock connectors), but they have not been accepted by the clinicians. They were too difficult to disconnect when treatments needed to be done. The tightness of connections caused extubations. Costs increased not only for the equipment itself but because two persons were needed when a disconnection was necessary for doing tasks that required sterile procedure.

Aside from improving in-service teaching and orientation of staff to the proper use of respirators, better monitoring of machine and patient, and close communication between manufacturer and users, this study of respirators concluded that no universal solution is likely. This is because staffs balance easy access to the airway, and related and necessary treatment, against considerations of cost, infection control, and patient comfort. In other words, the potential for errors associated with the disconnections is increased because of the multiple risks that must be considered by personnel.

In response to this study, another researcher, Janowski (1984a, 1984b), found further conditions that caused disconnections and still other risk reasons that mitigated against the use of antidisconnection devices, plus other conditions that triggered false alarms. Suggestions for preventing disconnections point to an increase in costs to the manufacturer or in costs to the hospital from making environmental and staff changes.

Considering the vast amount of machinery, drugs, and procedures that are used in concert, one can see that the risk-balancing judgments necessary for avoiding errors are rendered extremely difficult. For instance, in the Food and Drug study, a patient on an electrical rotating bed once became disconnected from the ventilator. Although the alarm sounded, it was mistaken for another alarm that indicated the electrocardiogram leads were detached—a frequent problem with this particular patient. In the confusion, the ventilator disconnection was not detected. Its cause was found to be the motion of the rotating bed. Unfortunately, as a result of this error, the patient died.

Human Sources of Error and Types of Errors

Human sources of error made by health workers include lack of skills—skills involving not only the knowledge necessary to make errorless judgments but also technical, manipulative skills necessary to carry out tasks. Both sets of skills are often based on experiential knowledge. Other sources of error consist of very human ones like carelessness or forgetfulness, being physically exhausted, or being distracted by other ongoing work or by personal pressures. Patients and families also may be sources of error. However, the instances of actually errorless work done by patients necessarily rests on professionals having made the patients' responsibilities explicit to them—for instance, what actions to avoid so as to prevent hazards. Patients' mis-assessments, because of their lack of knowledge or skill, inevitably lead to some damaging errors.

The types of errors pertain to basic work processes done at both the trajectory and task levels. At the trajectory level, errors include misdiagnosing an illness (such as through incomplete physical examinations or omitting pertinent laboratory tests), misassessing the hazards associated with illnesses in their various phases (usually underestimating and not taking preventive action), mismonitoring the unfolding trajectory, and misselecting the diagnostic, therapeutic, and palliative options either in kinds or combinations possible for the various trajectory phases. In addition, there is the mistiming (like waiting too long) of action associated with the perceived options for the unfolding trajectory. Also, since these carry many different risks, there may be a misbalancing of risks. The physician is largely responsible for the overall trajectory, and a physician error has far-reaching consequences. However, since the overall safety depends upon the work of many medical specialists and other health team members, errors made by others (such as a laboratory technician or nurse) may then lead to a physician's making a dangerous error in the trajectory management.

As noted in earlier chapters and further illustrated by the example of disconnections of ventilators, the safety requirements both at trajectory and task levels include those related to 1) clinical technical matters, 2) biography and identity of the patient, 3) comfort of the patient, 4) patient-staff and staff-staff interactions, and 5) composure of patient and staff. Since these are interrelated safety requirements, an omission or botching of a task related to one requirement may have negative consequences for another.

At the task level itself, there may be errors of misassessing, mismonitoring, and misrectifying the safety requirements set up to achieve an errorless task accomplishment. Other errors involve misaligning of a task sequence that stems either from misassessing, mismonitoring, or misrectifying the safety requirements, or from the occurrence of unexpected contingencies.

The organization of countless tasks carried out at various workplaces requires persons responsible for ensuring an errorless work flow. This is accomplished by allocating appropriate resources in accordance with changing safety requirements and the monitoring of potentials for errors, as well as by coordinating linkages between the work of various hospital departments, both for obtaining necessary services and goods and for rectifying organizational shortcomings. Errors can arise when inadequately prepared staff who are unable to handle properly the safety requirements are assigned to a task and/or when these staff jobs are not sufficiently monitored. The error potential is also raised by improperly maintained equipment, shortages of necessary supplies, unavailability of back-up resources (goods and personnel) as a safeguard for correcting errors, and poor interdepartmental relationships. Thus there are errors because of missupervision, too.

Finally, since both trajectory and task structure safety call for an immense amount of communication both laterally, as well as upward and downward among the various levels of workers, additional errors can originate from miscommunication. These may consist of omissions, unclear or ambiguous communications, or communications made to the wrong persons.

Properties of Error: Relevance to Error Management

Among the salient properties of errors are their 1) gravity, 2) discoverability, 3) predictability, 4) controllability, 5) rectifiability, and 6) cumulative impact on other errors. These properties are similar to those associated with danger/risk work (discussed in Chapter Three). The properties of danger and risk per se, and the anticipated properties of an error when made, are ordinarily both taken into account in the staff's error work.

For example, a given hazard may be highly predictable but fortunately preventable by a simple action. However, an omission of that action can have grave consequences. Furthermore, the rectification of this error can be difficult. So, staff will instead focus on doing preventive work. Error assessments in turn will involve assessing the properties of hazards without errors, their potentials for creating different kinds of error, the probable consequences, and the properties of errors once they occur. All of these assessments are used to determine the resources for monitoring and rectifying those conditions in order to prevent potential errors from occurring, as well as for matching resources in order to assess, monitor, and rectify errors once they occur.

After errors are committed, however, the assessments of hazard properties and error properties are taken into account when making judgments about culpability. An error will be judged harshly if its risk is grave but readily preventable—for example, forgetting to clamp off a chest drainage tube before disconnecting the drainage bottle. This error will cause lungs to collapse, which endangers not only the patients' respiratory status but cardiovascular status as well. Rectification for such a grave error may be difficult. On the other hand, errors that are difficult to assess and monitor are not so harshly judged. Also, various error properties are used by staff members to make normative judgments of each other or themselves: "He/she should have know better," or its opposite, "It could have happened to anybody."

A particularly confounding property of error is its potential discoverability. This property stems from the fact that the person who makes the error may not be observable when making it. And, in the absence of observability, the person who makes the error may not make the error public. A large proportion of actions of health workers are done when working alone. When an error is not actually observed in the making, then it may be discovered only through some unfavorable indicator (a patient's pscyhological or bodily reaction, a machine function, a laboratory test) that arouses the suspicion that an error has been committed. Of course, some errors go unrecognized. Others do not become apparent because they have no immediately associated indicators. Several days or even weeks may lapse before the indicators become apparent or are noticed. An example of such an error is when a physician overlooked a small bleeder during an operation and so the patient had a slow hemorrhage. Some errors do not become public because they are considered minor and readily rectified. Some errors are never discovered—or perhaps only years later are discovered either inadvertently through a medical examination that is not actually looking for it, or because a patient's symptoms take him/her to a physician who only then discovers the "old error."

Two striking features of hospital structure—that medical and nursing work involves many chains of tasks, which in turn involve many layers of workers—make particuarly difficult the quick determination of when, where, and by whom an error was made. Add to these structural conditions another set: 1) the complexity and ambiguity of many problematic trajectories whereby the making of errorless judgments is extremely difficult and 2) the complexity of the total arc of work. Thus, a retrospective discovery of error is not at all uncommon. Indeed, many patient case conferences can be described as retrospective error-analysis conferences. Recognizing that indeed one has made an error and then making the error public depends not only on the person's judgment at probable discovery of the error but also on a sense of moral and professional responsibility. Moreover, making the error public carries risks (to career, identity, patient-staff and staff-staff interactions), for both the person who made the error and the health team. If so, the balancing of these considerations may result in "covering up" and "sweeping under the rug."

Unless completely callous, every health worker takes into account the properties of error when an error is made or discovered. However, because personnel vary in their safety-error responsibilities and have different boundaries of work, they may also vary in their defining of the error properties. Effective error management depends upon the degree to which team members agree on the error dimensions, as well as their awareness of the others' definitions.

Organizational and Interactional Context of Assessing, Monitoring, and Rectifying Errors

The assessing and rectifying done when a clinical error is made or discovered is complex and often interactionally stressful for staff, patients, and families. The complexity stems from many interrelated factors. There are the consequences of an error for the patient and family, of course. There are also consequences for the person who made the error and for other workers who may have contributed to the mistake, as well as for the hospital itself. There is the issue of culpability and how this is to be managed. The rectifying not only must address the specific error as it affects the patient and the identities of staff involved but must prevent the error from reoccurring. Thereafter, the work must be monitored for its possible reoccurrence.

Thus, when an error is made, not one but many factors are assessed. These include, first of all, assessing the potential harm of the error to a patient. This is done to determine the monitoring and rectifying measures that must be instituted to control and reverse the known or potential damage. This type of assessment usually has first priority. Second, there is an assessing of how, when, why, and by whose actions the error occurred—that is, the circumstances associated with the error, the relevant series of events, and the kinds of misjudgments, carelessness, lack of manipulative skills and techniques, miscommunication or missupervision, and the miscoordination of work processes that may have been involved in the mistake. Third, there is an assessing of the risk consequences of the error for the error maker and for other personnel and hospital departments that may have contributed to the error. All of these factors are weighed and balanced to determine how to manage the person who made the error, as well as the kinds of monitoring and changes in work processes and in the division of labor needed to prevent its recurrence. The complexity of the management process will, of course, be shaped by the gravity of the error for the patient, the frequency of its occurrence, as well as the numbers and levels of workers and hospital departments involved.

Despite the anxiety generated among health workers when a bad error has been made, effective error work is often lacking. A major reason is that because the various implicated workers have different responsibilities and stakes in preventing or rectifying a given error, they are likely to weigh its risks differently; hence they disagree on solutions for preventing its occurrence or reoccurrence. Like rectification work, the prevention of error is a highly political process, for it requires much negotiation among many kinds and levels of workers.

Though standardized criteria may be used to assess errors, the decisions vary greatly concerning how to manage the person who makes an error. This is because personal values and experiences enter into the decisions—including the person's relationship to those making the assessment and his or her past clinical performances. Since everyone has committed errors, and indeed sometimes similar or identical ones, it is no wonder that personal experiences enter into judgments made both about the error makers and how they should be handled.

Such personal experiences are exemplified by the frequently uttered comment, when an error is made, "There but for the grace of God go I." Also, other staff will reveal their own errors in order to console the erring person. Thus, various degrees of tolerance exist for different kinds of errors. In general, however, readily preventable ones are harshly criticized. Severe criticism is directed against persons who commit errors during routine illness trajectories that result in severe damage or death. (An example would be a death brought about by complications of a hemorrhoidectomy, because the likelihood of complications was low and therefore everybody minimized the patient's complaints.) Indeed, the very routineness of a trajectory or task lends itself to error because then attention is focused more on other types of serious errors or because of the expectation that in such routine situations most workers will not make an error. Consequently, there is less monitoring of error.

To illustrate the variations of error that occur and the handling of the error maker—even when the errors are readily preventable—here is a mishap involving a nurse who gave an overdose of medication. The prescribed drug and the limits of its safe dosage were common knowledge because of its wide usage, so such a large overdose should have been recognized by her as unmistakably wrong. Her overdosing caused irreparable damage to the patient. The nurse's supervisor severely reprimanded her and assigned her to making a thorough study of the action of the implicated drug and of similar drugs, as well as their safe and proper administration. Another supervisor thought the nurse should have been fired outright, adding that even a first-year nursing student would not make such a stupid mistake.

Frequently, the existence of a potential error is well known to the staff, but its threat may not be remedied because of such reasons as cost or an inability to convince others of the need for attention. When the error does actually occur, then one hears remarks like "I knew it was going to happen; I kept complaining to the supervisor about this," or "Thank God, something is now going to be done about it."

The significant issue here is that although clinical safety has first priority for health professionals, errors actually play an important part in initiating attention and action that will establish the necessary work arrangements and criteria for assuring that work will be errorless. Given the bureaucratic complexity of acute care hospitals, a common if cynical view held by workers is that it takes an error to get any action.

Interactions involving errors are, in fact, probably the most difficult aspect of safety work. Interactional difficulties flow from the involvement of personal and professional identities, since judging an error often includes making negative judgments and criticisms about one's own and others' performances and competencies. There is also the onus of being directly or indirectly responsible for a mistake. Furthermore, the prevention of error requires interactions in order for staff members to assess each other's potentials, and, of course, this may require making negative judgments. Preventing and monitoring for error also involves overseeing others' performances. In addition to the supervising person observing them at work, the supervisor reminds them of probable errors that can be made, guiding their actions, or suggesting alternative courses of action. Then again, there is the pointing out of their actual errors. There are also interactions that take place around the reporting of errors— including one's own.

To make the matter still more complex, many difficulties attend the assessing of a given worker's error potential. These difficulties are derived from a paradox: even though educational and experiential standards are used to determine a worker's reliability, wide individual variations exist among workers, and these variations are often not immediately observable or assessable. Moreover, the assurance of errorless performance rests on other highly personal factors, such as a worker's conscientiousness and responsibility toward work, and the capacity to maintain composure under pressure or physical fatigue. Other important factors are the worker's self-awareness about his or her limitations of knowledge and experience, and willingness to reveal these limitations in order to prevent committing possible errors. In other words, moral character and integrity are involved. These highly personal considerations are often difficult to assess without extended observations and interactions. Under conditions of a shortage of nursing staff, relieved only by "floaters" and "temporary" workers, combined with high numbers of very acutely ill patients, tensions between the regular staff and relief workers may be high. There is then a lack of resources for properly assessing and observing the error potentials of the temporary workers, as well as resources for properly monitoring them. The errors then can be disastrous for patients.

Observations made to assess competence as well as error potential, especially while the work is actually still going on, must be handled so that the observed person does not become unduly nervous and upset. This necessity also may lead to error. Care must be taken so that those interactions will not be construed by the observed worker as a doubting of his or her competence or intelligence. In turn, the person overseeing the worker must minimize being perceived as a nag, or as being bossy or authoritarian.

The pointing out of errors indeed often requires great skill. Using sharp and loud comments such as "Don't you know any better!" can publicly humiliate the error maker, sometimes causing irreparable damage to future interactions. Then, when interactional errors are made, they too must be rectified in order to smooth future working relationships. Again, difficulties arise when errors are assessed differently. Making a big fuss about an error perceived by others as minor can damage the credibility of the overseer's supervisory skills and ability to separate the important from the unimportant.

Quite often the behavior in response to a mistake's being pointed out is used as a basis for making further judgments, not only about that worker's clinical competence but about personal characteristics regarded as related to his or her work.

Responses like not showing appropriate remorse for committing the error, or showing resentment, or blaming others for the error are often used for judging untrustworthiness or irresponsibility. Not infrequently these judgments may be accurate. However, the manner in which the error was pointed out (quietly versus loudly and angrily, or allowing or not allowing the error maker to explain the circumstances of the error, and so on) can determine the actual response of the reproved person.

The pointing out of impending or actual errors, and making suggestions to prevent future ones, can be done laterally or downward or upward in the personnel hierarchy. Interactional tensions can result when the suggestions are met with anger or sarcasm, or are ignored. Lower-status personnel are likely to be placed in vulnerable positions if they discover an error made by someone of higher status and then indicate this to him or her (Chavigny and Helm, 1982; Storlie, 1979).

The legal and interactional constraints that prevent an open discussion about errors, and the recording of them when there is a status difference, have been examined in a study of relationships between clinical pharmacists and physicians (Broadhead and Facchinetti, 1985). In this study, a new type of pharmacist—the clinical pharmacist—was involved with physicians and other health workers in direct patient care on the wards. The pharmacists acted as consultants, advising physicians on choices of drugs and their administration. This is an important function because of the explosion of new types of drugs in the last two decades that require very sophisticated knowledge to administer safely. These pharmacists also monitored drug use and caught physicians' prescription mistakes that might lead to serious consequences for patients.

The pharmacists were loath to document in the medical records questionable drug administration or errors. It was not uncommon in many hospitals for pharmacists to be prohibited from recording such items in patients' records, for it was thought this would increase the liability of the hospitals and their personnel. Documentation of the clinical activities was seen as quite a professional and legal threat. So, this posed dilemmas for the pharmacists. Without detailed and systematic documentation of their clinical activities, especially the catching of errors, pharmacists were unable either to demonstrate their contributions to patient care or to evaluate the adequacy of each other's clinical performances. They believed the avoidance of formal records did reduce the defensiveness of physicians and helped maintain good relationships with them. Good relationships were extremely important when the pharmacists desired acceptance in their new clinical role by the physicians. Interactionally, pharmacists felt compelled to call attention to apparent errors in a deferential manner that would not be interpreted as a questioning of physicians' expertise. They also avoided gestures that might be interpreted as "one-upmanship."

The delicacy of interactions and the sense of vulnerability felt by medical house staff when colleagues point out their errors is revealed in another study (Mizrath, 1984). When asked how they handle or tell a colleague if they saw a mistake or something wrong, they all expressed reticence to inform the other and said that the matter should be handled with great caution. They felt that it should be handled indirectly, very gently, with no reprimand or hassle or repercussion, in a joking manner, no rebuke or scolding, no tribunal, no yelling—all very polite and noncondemning, and diplomatic. The reason they gave for this was because "I am my own worst critic."

The above points to one of *the* most difficult aspects of error work: the regulation and surveillance of incompetents by their own colleagues. Although licensure regulations and ethical codes of practice govern the obligations of controlling incompetents, the sense of loyalty to one's own group, the sense of vulnerability that they themselves can make errors, and the hazards that accompany "whistle blowing"—all tend to discourage action for controlling incompetence (Bierig, 1980; Feliu, 1983; Mitchell, 1976; Regan, 1978; Storlie, 1979; Stelling and Bucher, 1973; Bosk, 1979; Freidson, 1976). Likewise, refusal to participate in certain acts that are judged as erroneous or involving wrongdoing sometimes takes great courage.

On the current nursing scene, concomitant with the women's rights movement, there is much concern with "assertiveness training'' (Donnelly, 1978; Fagin, 1975; Herman, 1978). Perusal of nursing journals quickly shows that many of the examples cited, and the areas where assertiveness is crucial, pertain to danger/safety issues and to error management, including handling discussions of others' errors with them.

One last point: the disclosures to patients and families about errors are extremely difficult for the staff to make. In fact, genuine disclosure seems seldom to be the case. More often than not, discussions with patients and families are couched in terms of ''unexpected complications'' or rationalized by thinking that to admit the mistake would destroy trust. Interactions become very strained when a patient or family suspects an error and malpractice suits lurk in the wings. Hence, avoidance and a conspiracy of silence usually prevail, among both staff and attending physicians. When discovery rather than disclosure occurs, or very great suspicion of error, then a malpractice suit or governmental review is likely. (The media event of Andy Warhol's unexpected death is an instance of this.) Occasionally a conscience-stricken insider can also tell or leak the secret, of course.

The ''Errorless Imperative'': The Need for Open Discussion

In hospitals today, the complicated medical technologies have understandably increased everyone's chances of making errors. As noted in the opening chapter, this, together with the fear of legal action, increases the drive among staff for the ''errorless imperative.'' But attempts to attain it are faced with all the dilemmas stemming from the many conflicting risk consequences.

In an interesting article wherein he bares his own mistakes, Dr. Hilfiker (1984) writes with anguish and honesty and quite possibly accuracy that the concern for legal liability, personal harm to one's own identity, and the very personal pain involved when an error is made tend to encourage denial and protectionism. Thus, he says, doctors hide their mistakes from patients, others, and even themselves. Mistakes become gossip and are only openly discussed in the courts. He adds that the heavy burden of infallibility demanded by both society and health professionals themselves poses an untenable problem. He calls for bringing mistakes out of the closet, adding that physicians need permission to admit their mistakes and to share them with their patients. There is probably much general truth to his self-observations, quite aside from his specific suggestions.

Everybody knows that mistakes are an everyday occurrence, since everyone has made and will continue to make them. Indeed, every action carries the potential for an error (Strauss, Fagerhaugh, Suczek, and Wiener, 1985). Yet there is a strong and unreasonable demand for infallibility. Mistakes are painful because one is confronted with one's own vulnerability. In many ways, mistakes by health professionals can be likened to the sense of failure and vulnerability that one feels when dealing with dying and death. Here again, although dying and death are faced daily by health professionals, nevertheless these topics or issues are not often discussed among them (Glaser and Strauss, 1965, 1968). Bringing death out of the closet has been a fairly recent development, the product of the so-called death and dying movement (Lofland, 1978; Charmaz, 1980).

Hence, caught as they are in the professional myth of infallibility or in the immediacy of legal liability risk, blame, and culpability, although mistakes are a central concern for all professionals, they are actually avoided as a topic of discussion or are only obliquely discussed. Interprofessional tensions and accusations about error, legal risk and error, and financial risk and error, dominate professional discourse. Formalized mechanisms, such as quality control review and peer review, are important to assure safety, yet the delicate interactional issues prevent much open discussion.

In the study by Mizrath (1984) of how 207 internist housestaff managed medical mistakes, it was found that these physicians had few opportunities to discuss errors openly. Hence they could not work out their sense of vulnerability and ambiguity, and often developed maladjusted modes of handling mistakes.

A nurse professor, who is a consultant to hospital nursing services, told us a story, expressing utter amazement. When she was a student back in the 1940s, a nurse making an error would fill out an "accident report." Some fifteen years later this form was called an "incident report." Now, in the 1980s, she has found that several hospitals use a "variance report." Obviously the latter term refers to variations from accepted standards of performance. This story indicates the growing concern of hospital administrators with the legal implication of staff errors. Such terms as *variance report* obfuscate the real and pressing need for open discussion, and their use is not unlike calling lying "disinformation."

There is a pressing need for staff opportunities to discuss error critically and openly, to gain group support, and to find ways to improve error management and interaction. There is also a need for educational programs so that health professionals can find effective ways for teaching students to cope with this very difficult issue.

Summary

Error management was examined in the context of today's work situations, particularly the legal issues that increasingly affect hospital work. Error work—the work of managing errors—was then discussed, including measures to prevent errors as well as to monitor, assess, and rectify them. Some of the difficulties in doing this include the complexity of technologies interacting with the problematic character of some chronic illnesses. Tracheal-machine disconnections were used to illustrate this point. We then turned to consideration of the human sources of error and types of errors. The latter occur in relation to work processes on both the trajectory and the task levels, and they include misassessing, mismonitoring, mistiming, misbalancing of risks, misrectifying, and miscommunication. We next discussed salient properties of errors and some of their consequences for staff strategies as well as for staff interactions. In the final two sections of this chapter, we discussed the complicated organizational and interactional context within which error management occurs and then argued the need for much more open discussion of errors within hospitals and with patients and their families.

6

〜〜〜〜〜〜〜〜〜〜〜〜〜〜〜〜〜〜〜〜〜〜〜〜〜〜〜〜

Recognizing and Enhancing
Patients' Contributions
to Safety Management

Thus far, our discussion of clinical hazard has focused primarily on the professional staff. However, the patients, and often their families, are also busily engaged in safety work; they are very much involved in preventing, monitoring, assessing, and rectifying hazards. This is because it is their bodies and selves that are being endangered. They are often aware that if they do not watch carefully, they may suffer the consequences of staff's errors. The duality of their being both sources of danger and objects of potential risks poses particular difficulties for both the patients and staff in carrying out their safety responsibilities.

Patients as Safety Workers

In the acute care hospital setting, tasks performed by patients often go unnoted by the staff, because much of their work is not defined as "work" (Strauss, Fagerhaugh, Suczek, and Wiener, 1981, 1982; Stepter, 1981). Staff members regard their own work as professionalized and linked with their occupational titles. By contrast, the tasks performed by patients are neither professionalized nor occupationally linked. So the idea of patients as workers is essentially nonexistent, although implicitly their work is often recognized—and certainly utilized. The prevailing concept held by health professionals that patients are

140

"clients" or "consumers" to whom services are rendered, or "clients" whose "needs" are to be met, connotes passive persons who do not actively work in their own behalf (Chang, 1980; Conway-Rutowsky, 1982). Various social scientists have criticized this passive view of patients and have called for more control by patients over their own care (Johnson, 1977; Jobling, 1976; Stacey, 1976). However, they do not analyze patients' work quite as we do, and not in the crucial context of chronic illness prevalence.

When patients refuse to perform certain tasks, then frequently the staff is likely to refer to them as "uncooperative," "irresponsible," or "recalcitrant." Such terms often point to some personality factor underlying the refusal. Yet, imbedded in these terms is actually the expectation that patients are held accountable for carrying out certain tasks, for patients play an active role in the division of labor during their care. First of all, unless very acutely ill, they are expected to do the major part of their own bodily hygiene work (bathing, brushing teeth, and so on). When health professionals perform procedures "on" the patients, the latter are expected to do their own work of not moving and maintaining a certain body position, not yelling (as this would upset the professionals' performance), and maintaining composure even though the procedures may be painful. Or they must work at ambulating after surgery even though very weak and frightened. All of this work requires extending much energy, effort, and sometimes much courage.

In the hospital context, then, the patient is a very important part of a division of labor. In getting work done, bundles of tasks must be ordered sequentially and/or simultaneously. While the staff is doing necessary tasks, the patient must sequentially and/or simultaneously perform other tasks in order to get the work done. If the patient's tasks are not performed, then the work may be done improperly. Some work may even require that a patient do the major task, such as deep breathing to prevent respiratory infections. Other work may involve the alignment of tasks performed by several people, including the patient, as in carrying out complex medical or nursing procedures.

In acute care hospitals today, since most patients are suffering through acute phases of chronic illnesses, they have had much experience in managing their own illnesses. Frequently, their frustration or anger can result in overt conflict with the staff when the patients believe—whether rightly or wrongly—that staff members know less than they do about the immediate illness condition and what should be done about it. Far less obvious but probably more important, however, is their covert and unobtrusive work that goes unnoted by the staff. Of course, some of the work may be noted, but its importance discounted.

Because patients are largely responsible for their own care at home during nonacute phases, the current emphasis on teaching self-care to them within the hospitals represents an effort to teach them to take responsibility for successfully managing their own care. Since today lives can be extended by use at home of a variety of complex technologies—such as kidney dialysis and respiratory machines—then it is reasoned that patients and families must be taught to be skilled technicians. Then, of course, their work is so visible that it is genuinely recognized. Also, the current emphasis on self-care is also motivated in part by concern over reduction of the costs of health care. For instance, kidney dialysis at home is far less costly than at health care settings (Warner and Kolff, 1977). Ironically, the decreased public costs of home care rest on the unpaid efforts of the ill and their families.

Types of Patient Safety Work

The division of labor between the professionals and hospitalized patients will, of course, depend on professional, legal, and jurisdictional limits imposed on the professionals. It will also be influenced by staff and lay ideologies: whether they believe patients are important collaborators in their care or passive followers of the professionals' dictates. The division of labor will also vary according to kinds and quality of the bundles of tasks involved in the trajectory phases and miniphases, amount of skill and attention required, amount of coordination of tasks done by the various workers, and so on.

There are several types of work engaged in by patients. First, some work is done in tandem with the staff's work. Patients give urine, then the staff sends it to the laboratory for testing. Patients obey commands to take certain body positions in conjunction with the staffs' medical and nursing procedures. Second, some work by patients is supplementary to the staff's, such as maintaining composure in the face of nursing procedural tasks. Third, the work may substitute for the staff's work, such as monitoring a bodily reaction to a medical or nursing intervention. This work may be explicitly delegated by the staff, implicitly understood by the patient, negotiated between them, or volunteered by the patient. Fourth, patients do work that they believe is necessary, such as monitoring for potential error by or incompetence of the staff. Quite often this work is invisible to the staff. Fifth, patients may rectify staff errors, either by directly doing the rectifying themselves or reporting—or complaining—to the proper authorities. Sixth, they do work that only the patient can do, such as giving highly personalized information about allergic reactions to certain drugs or about illnesses that pose problems in managing the main illness for which they were hospitalized. Furthermore, a large part of their additional work, usually done with little assistance from the staff, is coping with identity problems precipitated by the illness— for instance, struggling with disfigurement or the fear of impending death.

When clinical dangers and risks are anticipated and the work involves patients' cooperation, then their safety work is made explicit by staff. When an intervention is highly risky, as in open-heart surgery, the staff tends to be very specific about the expected safety tasks. They are very well aware that patients must be persuaded to do these tasks because much effort must be exerted by the patients under difficult and painful circumstances. There are also standardized patient instruction forms apprising patients about what to expect in difficult types of diagnostic tests and the work they must do for a successful outcome (take no foods after midnight, take a laxative to clean the bowels, and so on).

Mutual Assessment and
Misassessment by Patient and Staff

Since both patient and staff can be sources of hazards, both assess and monitor each other's hazard potentials. Staff try to assess medical sophistication and other personal attributes (intelligence, alertness, emotional status, and so on) to determine if a patient can be responsible for required safety tasks. Also, their assessments determine if information about bodily reactions is reliable and believable. Patients, in turn, assess and monitor the risk potentials of staff members: whether they are competent, reliable, and trustworthy. Although the cues utilized by both parties can be accurate, interaction between patient and staff can lead to discounting of each other's assessments. For example, a patient who develops a reputation as a "whiner" may face difficulty in getting the personnel to accept an accurate assessment of a bodily reaction. Likewise, if the staff is considered incompetent by the patient, he or she may discount their information and directives. A tricky, silent game is played wherein both parties size up each other and attempt to present themselves in such a manner that they are accepted as reliable, competent, and believable (Goffman, 1959).

Patients are at a great disadvantage in making educated judgments about the staff's competence. Thus, the patients often collaborate with each other in making assessments. Patient-patient and patient-kin conversations are replete with assessments of staff competency. "Boy, Nurse X sure knows her stuff," "You got to watch Miss Jones," or "I feel worse today because I don't think Miss X knows how to do the treatments."

More often than not, patients are also at a disadvantage because they have neither the experience nor the medical knowledge—and often recognize this—to make accurate judgments about hazards. However, some do become quite expert. For example, because kidney dialysis patients have treatments several times a week, they develop expertise not only in assessing staff competence but in monitoring both the treatments and their bodies while on dialysis.

Patients' assessing and monitoring activities are often based on very personal experiences with illness that are not known to the staff. These experiences color the patients' priorities, making some hazardous items quite important, though others may be actually or equally more important "medically." For instance, one man had developed an infection at the intravenous puncture site during his previous hospitalization, so he assessed and closely monitored the personnel who were now doing the procedure—whether they washed their hands, and so on. He even refused to have anyone he judged as clumsy or physically untidy carry out the procedure. The staff, in turn, thought he was "being a bit fussy" and "a little on the paranoid side."

Patients' refusals to have certain personnel do the treatments, their requests for changes in nurses assigned to them, and their pointed suggestions about how to do a procedure are efforts to prevent or rectify what they assess as potential hazards to their clinical comfort or identity safety. Because their actions involve reassignment of work and thereby upset the ward's work order, anger may be generated in the staff members. Also, such actions are seen by the staff as an assault on their identities, bringing into question their competence. Recognizing this, the patients are likely to remain silent because they do not wish to endanger interactions with the staff. Sometimes family members act on patients' behalf at the expense of causing strain between themselves and staff.

A central problem in getting a better match between the respective assessments is that generally each applies different criteria. The personnel tend to rely on technical measures, whereas patients rely on their own bodily reactions and sensations, mainly their pain and other discomforts. Those indicators are highly subjective, and in addition many discomforts are very ambiguous. The ambiguity is partly due to there being several kinds of discomforts and partly because their sources may or may not be related to illness. (This point will be discussed in greater detail in the next chapter.)

Examples of Patients' Safety Work

As we have noted, patients engage in assessing, monitoring, preventing, rectifying, balancing, and weighing the multiple hazards. Even within a given episode, all of these subtypes of safety work may be involved. For example, here is one that took place when an intravenous (IV) ran out because the nurses forgot to monitor the IV. This occurred on the first postoperative day. Both because of the patient's previous hospitalization and her friends' hospitalizations, she was acutely aware that intravenous mismonitoring would require another uncomfortable vein puncture.

> I wasn't about to get another needle puncture because of a nurse forgetting to check the IV. During the night I kept turning the light on to check the IV. But I had so much pain (from surgery) I had to have a shot to relieve the pain. But the shot made me sleepy even though I tried to stay awake. I fell asleep. And wouldn't you know it, the IV ran out! The nurses were short-staffed, and there were a number of very sick patients so they forgot to check the IV. Then the only registered nurse on duty seemed so unsure of herself about restarting another IV. I tried to bargain to hold off the IV until morning, but the nurse felt I needed the IV. I was in a quandary, whether to refuse to let her do it—and she was really a very nice person. She was very apologetic about not watching the IV and was very upset. I felt sorry for her. Then I thought I've got veins that are really easy to get at—so I've been told. So I decided to let her try, but it would be for only two stabs. Fortunately she got into the vein OK. I was so relieved.

Her story illustrates the many kinds of safety work engaged in during just one episode. Thus, she monitored the IV to prevent a potential body discomfort risk, assessed the condition of her veins and the competence of the nurse to do a safe and discomfort-free puncture, and also sought an alternative to getting a puncture. Based on her assessments she decided what she would risk but set the risk limit at "two stabs." Also, she weighed and balanced the nurse's composure against her own. Finally, her story illustrates how organizational contingencies, such as staffing and other work, strongly affect safety work.

This particular patient also worked hard at preventing discomforts caused by an incompatible analgesic. During a previous hospitalization she had become extremely nauseated from Demerol (meperidine hydrochloride), but not from morphine sulfate. To prevent a mistake being made by the staff, she reported the drug incompatibility to a nurse when being admitted to the hospital, and to the medical house staff, the attending surgeon, and the anesthesiologist during the presurgery workup. In addition, before accepting a pain drug injection, she checked to make sure that she was not getting the incompatible drug.

Another complex example: a patient was admitted to the same unit for a repetition of a risk-laden neurological surgery. He reminded the staff that he had developed a postoperative infection during his previous hospitalization, which he thought was because of staff negligence, a complication that extended his hospitalization. So, during this second hospitalization he participated vigorously in the work of preventing respiratory complications. In addition, previously he had developed a backache from having to maintain the sitting position important for success of the surgery—a backache that persisted for months after the surgery. To decrease the chances of a potential backache, he brought to the hospital special foam pads and pillows, with which he had experimented and had found decreased his discomfort. For weeks prior to the surgery he engaged in back exercises to prevent a backache reoccurrence. He also attempted to negotiate for earlier ambulation than during the previous hospitalization, in order to prevent a reoccurrence of the backache. However, he was unsuccessful in convincing his physician, who judged this activity would compromise the neurosurgery. The nurses and the house staff thought the attending physician was being unduly cautious but went along with his decision. At first the patient cooperated, but his backache recurred. Codeine was prescribed for the surgical pain and the backache, but this drug constipated him. Family members brought in extra fruit to relieve the constipation. Finally, when he felt stronger, he would stand on the side of the bed, for he felt this relieved the backache. He requested heat for his back to relieve the backache, but this gave little relief. Nurses and house staff were sympathetic to his plight but would not negotiate on his behalf with the attending physician for earlier ambulation. They did not wish to challenge the physician, a powerful and important person on the medical staff. Of course, tests were done to determine the cause of the backache, but they were negative. The patient was fully aware of the physician's reasons for caution about early ambulation and tried to cooperate. After it seemed to him that his surgical recovery was on schedule, and since his backache had increased because of having to maintain a sitting position in bed, he would sneak out of bed and walk. He assured the nurses that he would take full responsibility should they be scolded by the physician for allowing him to countermand the orders.

This case illustrates the amount of work and negotiation engaged in by the patient, both before and during the hospitalization, in order to prevent and rectify risks. It also illustrates how patients and staff can vary in risk priorities, for this patient also assessed the surgical risks in relation to the discomfort and pain risks caused by the backache. We can also see that staff and patients can differ in what risks they take into account when solving a problem. Fortunately, in this case the risks were not life-threatening. However, when risks are multiple and potentially life-threatening, and divergent hazard priorities are held by the patient and staff (and even families), then effective safety work can be rendered extremely difficult.

While the patients are in the hospital, families do an immense amount of safety work. Often this is also invisible to the staff. For instance, they act as safety watchdogs. Here is an illustration of this point. A medically sophisticated relative (a nurse) of a patient correctly assessed a patient as being in potentially hazardous electrolyte imbalance. The staff discounted the assessment as reflecting an overanxious nurse-relative. At first she used gentle persuasion, but finally she resorted to legal threat in order to get the hazardous condition rectified. After its rectification, the researcher made a remark to her about her being a "regular watchdog" for the patient. She agreed that was an apt term, adding that one has to "yip, yap, and bark a lot" to be heard. Yet in these professional-kinsmen encounters considerable interaction skills by the kin are required to assure a relative's safety. The difficulties encountered even by those who are medically sophisticated kin—or are professionals themselves—emphasize the difficulties that unsophisticated kin may encounter in trying to assure a relative's safety.

Transmission and Exchange of Information

In recent years, expectations by patients and their families for fuller information exchange and disclosure concerning hazards has increased, in part because of the consumer movement (as reflected in such issues as "patients' rights," "informed consent," "patients' access to medical records") and the growth of self-help groups (Gartner and Riessman, 1984). These trends reflect an effort to increase participation in health care services and to reorder the power imbalance, most particularly patient-physician relationships, from submissive patient versus supreme physician authority to a more equitable balance. The reordering of patient-professional relationships has been legally mandated by changes in both common and statutory law. The American Hospital Association's Patient's Bill of Rights sets forth the extent of a patient's privileges but also makes clear the legal precedence of the hospital's responsibility to patients. "Informed consent" establishes the principle that physicians must disclose all relevant information of hazards and risks that a reasonable person would need in order to make an intelligent decision about the physician's proposals for intervention. Informed consent has been accepted with varying degrees of reluctance by professionals (Taylor and Kelner, 1987), particularly by physicians, since the major responsibility of disclosing information usually rests with them.

Informed consent has been criticized on various grounds (Wiener, Fagerhaugh, Strauss, and Suczek, 1980). First, information given is not necessarily received. Studies are cited demonstrating barriers to patients' realistic understanding—

lack of education, lack of interest, high anxiety level, and status differences between physicians and patients. One study found that only high-status patients who ask appropriate questions will indicate mistrust, and that others will assume there is an obligation of compliance if they are to maintain an amicable relationship with physicians (Gray, 1975). Another ground for criticism has to do with the psychological effects of providing information to patients, with the side effect of potentially increased anxiety. A third ground for criticism relates to the complex intertwining of informed consent with the legal protectionism of professionals. Critics argue that the intent of informing patients and protecting their rights has turned into professional preoccupation with the "malpractice menace," so that in part patients' rights are de-emphasized. The practice of "defensive medicine"—delaying the use of potent drugs, encouraging excessive laboratory and x-ray tests, or fostering unnecessary consultations—may expose patients to additional hazards and/or increase health care costs. Critics further argue that standards of informed consent are neither what a reasonable doctor would tell a patient nor what a reasonable patient would want to know. Additionally, they argue that the demands of informed consent may result in information overload for the patient who needs time to digest and discuss information (Alfidid, 1975). Quite often, informed consent is reduced more to patients consenting rather than patients being informed. As Annas has pointed out, frequently there is more disclosure on the part of the physician than understanding on the part of the patient (Annas, Glantz, and Katz, 1977).

Patient-staff interaction concerning information about hazards and disclosure by staff is far from easy. It requires much interactional skill and much biographical information about patients and families. Moreover, disclosure may be complicated by the ambiguity attending many illnesses and their associated technological interventions. In fact, debates among professionals about safe options, and when and how they are to be applied, are common occurrences. In addition, when illnesses are multiple, as often today, several specialists and experts are involved—so that the primary physicians may well be reduced to laypersons in relation to other specialists, perhaps deferring to them more blindly than is warranted.

The ambiguity of hazards can also become the basis of misunderstanding between patient and professionals. For example, the physician may hesitate to disclose information because the situation is ambiguous or requires further data, but the patient then construes the silence as deliberate evasion. Or when the ambiguity is disclosed, because the patient is directly involved in the hazard, the patient may then press for nonambiguous answers that the professional cannot actually deliver. Persistent patients who press for nonambiguous answers can pose difficult interactional problems.

An instructive account can be found in *A Coronary Event* (Halberstam and Lesher, 1976) by Michael Halberstam, who treated the patient, and Stephen Lesher, who was in his thirties when he had his first myocardio-infarct. The two authors wrote of their mutual experiences: how they experienced and perceived the many events, each other, and the hospital personnel. This patient, an investigative newspaper reporter (then very involved in the Watergate investigation), who was skilled in gathering information, aggessively sought information. He used such tactics as checking out the validity and reliability of information, by asking the same question framed differently of the same doctor or different doctors and by confronting doctors with inconsistent information received from one or another of them. The information received from them he compared with information got from his reading of medical literature and from talking with other cardiac patients. Then he confronted the staff with treatment variations and inconsistencies of medical information. His misunderstandings and misconstruings of information were frequent. Information given by professionals in the early phase of hospitalization, while the danger prognosis was still unclear, was doggedly pursued by this patient, even though his physical condition had changed during later phases of his illness. Information and responses from the attending physician meant to relieve his anxiety were interpreted as evasive or patronizing. Seemingly innocuous information from residents and interns was used against the attending physician or blown out of proportion. All of this earned the patient an unfavorable reputation and resulted in the staff's meting out subtle and not-so-subtle punishment for his "uncooperativeness." Eventually his physician and he were able to gain mutual trust, but not without considerable interactional tension. The tactics used by this patient-author to obtain information and to establish its reliability and validity are not dissimilar to those used by other patients, only differing in degree of sophistication and interactional style. Few patients act as aggressively and brashly as he did.

The case of this coronary patient ended happily, but a contrasting case is highlighted by Robert and Peggy Stinson's account in an article entitled "On the Death of a Baby" (Stinson and Stinson, 1979). They were parents of a premature infant who was at the extreme margin of human viability. He was placed in a respirator against parental wishes and consent, and cared for in a neonatal intensive care unit. He died after months of heroic efforts to save him, efforts that had resulted in a long list of iatrogenic afflictions. The ultimate end saw the parents having great bitterness and expressing great anger against the medical staff. Their tragic account describes the tremendous difficulties faced in obtaining information from the medical staff and being forced to find information on their own at the medical school library. Attempts to get information from the staff and to participate in treatment decisions were rebuffed. In addition, their efforts were harshly judged as "not wanting the child," "hostile," "emotionally fragile," and so on through a litany of pejorative terms.

The contrast between the two cases (the coronary event and the dying infant) can, of course, be explained away as due entirely to differences in sensitivity and humanity of the respective medical staffs, for the physician in the coronary event had considerable sensitivity toward his patient, in contrast to the insensitivity of the neonatal critical care medical staff. However, the two cases can surely also be analyzed in terms of conditions affecting the two trajectories in relation to hazards and their relevance to information disclosure.

If we further compare the two cases described above, we find first of all that they differed widely in terms of their medical-historical time frames. The application of high technology in coronary care had been in use for some time, partly as a result

of extensive financial support for federal research and development in coronary care technology during the 1960s. In spite
of many ambiguities in the coronary situation, the hazards of
care could be more accurately assessed and controlled than in
the neonatal intensive care situation. However, the application
of high technology in neonatal care and development of neonatal
intensive care units have been later developments, so that in
1976 (when the described event occurred) much of the technology
there was fraught with unknowns and uncertainties. Then, too,
as is characteristic of pioneering medical situations, the desire
to find answers and solutions to technical medical problems tends
to foster an experimental stance by the medical staff at the expense of the patient's (and kin's) pain and suffering.

There is another point of difference between the two cases.
Because the coronary trajectory was limited to a single illness,
information exchange and disclosure could be handled by only
one physician, a cardiologist. The infant's case involved several
body systems and therefore involved several specialists along
with interns and residents who were rotating through the intensive care unit. The ability to extend lives today, as on the
intensive care nursery (ICN) brings with it a high probability
for trajectories to go so awry that they become a "cumulative
mess" (Fagerhaugh and Strauss, 1977; Strauss, Fagerhaugh,
Suczek, and Wiener, 1985).

Aside from these two cases in general, it is safe to say that
the ease and dis-ease of disclosure by staffs and their giving of
information to patients and families are related partly to the
degree that hazard dimensions originating from various sources
during the evolving trajectory phases can be accurately assessed,
anticipated, and controlled. The more problematic the danger
and risk dimensions, their sources, and the associated trajectory phases, the greater then are the variabilities—variabilities
both in assessment and in hazards being balanced differently
by the patient and the staff, as well as within the staff itself.
Moreover, anxiety and stress are high. All of this fosters misunderstanding and misconstruing of information by patients and
families, and the misjudging of appropriateness (what, how, and
when) of information disclosure.

Making Disclosures: Variations and Consequences

A central problem in information disclosure and exchange about risk is the differences among health professionals in their assessments of risks, as well as in their balancing the consequences of disclosure. They also differ in their views of the ethical values of disclosure. Decisions are made about (1) the extent of disclosure (from withholding to total openness), (2) the kinds of information disclosed, (3) the interactional approach (minimizing or emphasizing the risks to the patient or the degree of persuading or manipulating of the appropriate information, and (4) the appropriateness of timing. These decisions are based not only on the overall assessment of potential clinical risks but on the balancing of risk consequences. Recall the balancing matrix of risk consequences discussed in Chapter Four, concerning what is disclosed by staff. What is disclosed and how is based on such balancing. Staff opinions can vary widely not only about how disclosure consequences may impact on the patient's bodily management but also on the patient's behavior. Staff members also balance consequences for future patient-staff and staff-staff interactions, and for their own identities. They can differ in their moral judgments about "good and bad," "should and ought," such matters as when is it permissible to withhold information (as about dying), and what is considered deception.

Usually disclosures are made by a single staff member. However, that person does not normally inform other personnel of the disclosure, and seldom is there any ensuing discussion with the patient. Patient-staff and staff-staff interactional difficulties with patients and other staff members can result when the latter are not aware of the items of disclosure or the basis for the disclosure action. For instance, in the case of Mrs. Price (Chapter Two), the ward staff as a group tended to minimize the harm to her kidney from the radiation treatment of her stomach. They reasoned that the treatment was the wisest option for that particular phase of the illness course. The radiologist who did the treatment, unaware of the basis for the ward staff's action, informed the patient of the kidney hazard. The patient interpreted this as more serious than previously she had been led to believe. Already reluctant to undergo the radiation treatment, she began to resist the therapy even more vigorously.

Nurses feel particularly vulnerable in disclosure interactions. Unaware of the nature of the physician's disclosure discussion with a patient, the nurses' responses may run counter to the physician's disclosure information. The result is an unduly upset patient. Of course, there is also the potential risk for nurses of being accused of interference with the patient-physician relationship—or still worse, interfering with the sacred and legalized treatment domain of the physician. Each infraction could constitute unprofessional behavior. This was the situation in the Tuma case (Tuma, 1977), in which a nurse discussed alternative options to cancer chemotherapy, without consulting the physician. To avoid these potential negative consequences, the nurses' usual approach is first to explore the patient's understanding of the physician's disclosure discussion. Then they assist the patient in airing any fears and anxieties. Hopefully, such a discussion will help the patient find ways of raising unanswered questions with the physician. Of course, a nurse may elect to discuss this further with the physician.

In short, a tremendous amount of intrateam exchange of information is necessary in order for staff members to become aware of each other's differing concerns about the consequences of disclosing hazards to patients. This exchange of information is critical for disclosure interactions to be handled sensitively and to prevent patients from feeling avoided or depersonalized.

When patients believe the information offered by staff is inadequate, they attempt to establish the validity and the reliability of information received. Of course, as do health professionals themselves, they rely on the usual staff expertise hierarchy (nurse, intern, resident, attending physician, specialist, chief of staff) to determine the degree of its reliability. In addition, they closely watch how professionals present the information, especially their accompanying facial expressions and body languages. "I know I'm over the hump because today the doctor smiled when he said, 'You're coming along fine.' Two days ago he said the same thing, but his face was grimmer." Or, "I am wondering if indeed the risks are not so serious; he [doctor] seemed so circumspect." Patients search for approachable health personnel to get answers, as quite often do their acquaintances

and relatives. Indeed, during the course of our research, patients would sometimes ask us if we were familiar with a given
technology or procedure, or with the physician's reputation. In
the search for validity and reliability, nurses are frequently ques-
tioned, partly because of their availability. A nurse may hesitate,
answering "You'll have to ask your doctor," for fear of the consequences of the anger of a physician who does not believe in
genuine disclosure. In essence (in patient safety work terms),
ineffective disclosure interaction by the staff increases patients'
information-seeking work.

Critics point out that in spite of professional efforts to share
information, the Aesculapian authority (power based on physician's expertise, the patient's faith in the physician, and the belief
that the physician has almost mystical powers) (Siegler and Osmond, 1973) continues to be strong. In consequence, truly
equitable patient-professional interactional approaches are very
difficult to achieve. Even for medically sophisticated persons,
to oppose traditional authority is very difficult. This difficulty
has been described vividly by Beatrice Kalisch (1975), a prominent and medically knowledgeable nurse, in her account of
coming to a decision about having surgery. She further points
out that the physicians' exercising of the Aesculapian authority,
as is most frequently singled out, is the villain, but that nurses,
too, are involved in maintaining its rule.

Patient Teaching and Patient Advocacy

As already discussed in the previous chapter, a vast amount
of information must be exchanged about a wide range of information so that patients can effectively participate in safety work.
Currently much of this exchange takes the form of "patient
teaching." To this end, over the past decade pamphlets, books,
audiovisual and booklet teaching aids have proliferated. In large
institutions, departments solely concerned with patient teaching
have developed. There are informal, individualized, and group
teaching sessions of patients. Frequently these follow a planned
lesson approach where the content is well defined. In essence,
these teaching approaches are usually formulated in terms of
a teacher-learner model. Although these efforts are commend-

able and should be continued, there are limitations to this model. It tends to emphasize a hierarchical relationship that may hinder more equitable sharing (Engel, 1978; Strauss, Fagerhaugh, Suczek, and Wiener, 1982). Where there is a hierarchical relationship, the teacher role is likely to prevent the teacher from gaining full understanding of the patient's true perceptions— so necessary in the collaborative effort of managing an illness (Jacobs, 1981).

In a trend accompanying the consumer rights movement, professionals have shown a growing interest in incorporating advocacy roles to improve patient care. This trend is popular among nurses. Their interest seems related in part to the caring role traditionally associated with nursing. Their interest is also based on their humanistic concerns about protecting patients from the depersonalizing effects of hospitals. They are concerned with the deception of patients in health facilities and the need for protecting patients' rights (Donahue, 1982). Patient advocacy is popular among nurse theorists in their efforts to define nurses' professional roles. It is also supported by the American Nurses Association (American Nurses Association, 1979; Chapman and Chapman, 1975; Simms and Lindbergh, 1979).

A variety of notions have been proposed and applied about the advocacy role relative to the nurse's relationship with the patient, the profession, and the health care institutions. The identified responsibilities include acting as a counselor to patients, helping them maintain autonomy about their care, assisting them in gaining access to information, educating them about making informed treatment choices, helping them to exercise their rights, and protecting them from any actions of health care givers judged to be inappropriate or harmful. In essence, the nurse's responsibilities range from being a supportive counselor to taking a more active adversarial role (Abrams, 1978; Donahue, 1982; Flaherty, 1981; Jenny, 1979; Kohnke, 1980; Oberle, 1982; Smith, 1980). Consequently, there are conflicts with physicians, the profession, and the hospital. These conflicts have resulted in advocates losing licenses to practice, and even jobs (Oberle, 1982; Flaherty, 1981; Smith, 1980). The conflicts have resulted in hostilities arising between nurses and physicians, nurse administrators, other nurses, as well as between physicians and patients.

Efforts are being made to establish guidelines for delineating those situations when particular cautions are necessary and for finding those strategies that will effectively protect the patient and at the same time will avoid conflicts of interest (Curtin and Flaherty, 1982; Zussman, 1982).

In the context of our safety discussion, the nurses' patient-advocacy role is designed to find ways of assisting patients to do their safety work more efficiently and of assisting them in balancing and weighing the consequences of risks associated with the medical treatment, as well as in preventing and rectifying harmful situations. In doing this, nurses—ironically— must assess and balance the consequences of taking on this advocacy role.

Summary

Patients are very much involved in many types of safety work, but their work often goes unrecognized by the health personnel. Patients and staff mutually assess each other as potential sources of hazard, but their assessments can be based on differing criteria that also go unrecognized. Consequently, misunderstandings are very likely to ensue. Examples of patients' (and families') safety work were given to illustrate these points. Also, various difficulties encountered in transmission and exchanges of information by both patients and staff were discussed, with particular emphasis on "informed consent." Conflicts involving staff with staff and patient with staff over information transmission and exchanges are in part related to how staff members vary in their balancing of the consequences of risk disclosure. Although efforts are made to improve information exchange through "patient teaching," the teacher-learner model that lies behind these efforts does limit the development of a more equitable and collaborative sharing of information. The nurses' patient-advocacy role for improving patient care also reflects that the difficulties encountered stem from the conflicts over assessing risk consequences by the various health personnel.

7

҂ҫ҂ҫ҂ҫ҂ҫ҂ҫ҂ҫ҂ҫ҂ҫ҂ҫ҂ҫ҂ҫ҂ҫ҂ҫ҂ҫ҂ҫ҂ҫ҂ҫ

Relieving the Physical
and Psychosocial Discomfort
of Patients

What used to be called traditional *caring* or the giving of *tender loving care* is work that deals with the management of many physical and subjective pains and discomforts suffered by patients. Since these sufferings are closely related to their social and physical identities, patients' and families' accusations of hospital staff's negligence, incompetence, and dehumanized care most often revolve around pains and discomforts that they believe have been mismanaged. There are two separate components of caring: *comfort work* and what we shall refer to as *sentimental work.*

Comfort work is embedded in the total clinical work, since in doing any clinical intervention on the patient, inflicted discomforts and psychological dis-ease associated with the intervention must—or at least should—be managed. While comfort is essential for clinical safety, it also constitutes an important safety work in and of itself.

In spite of recognition by health professionals that this is so, there are problems in actually ensuring that comfort care is given safely. In the first place, much uncertainty is associated with the very subjective phenomena of pain and discomfort. These phenomena can arise from multiple sources: from the disease, as symptoms of clinical dangers; from the staff, in the form of inflicted discomforts (perhaps hazardous) when performing various procedures on the patient; from various diagnostic and therapeutic measures, in the form of side effects or complications; from mismanaged patient-staff interactions, in the form of wounded sensibilities; or from normal, everyday bodily activities associated with eating, sleeping, mobilizing, and so on. Thus, pain and discomfort can be indicators of clinical dangers or risk consequences of mismanaged clinical, identity, or interactional safety work. This ambiguity poses problems in assessment. Given the array of pains and discomforts arising from multiple sources, together with their subjectivity, there is a likelihood of disagreement over priorities between patient and staff as well as among staff members. Second, the intensity of the clinical safety work competes with comfort safety. The complexity of the clinical safety task structure and the many contingencies that can disarticulate this work, along with the high number of patients with problematic illnesses, result in immediate clinical hazards taking priority over long-term discomfort hazards. Third, because of the subjectivity of pain and discomfort, patients are important participants in this work. However, the ambiguity associated with pain and discomfort, together with the differences between staff and patients about discomfort priorities, pose problems for patients in doing this work.

Sentimental work or the humanistic concern for patients' psychological suffering, is usually referred to by health professionals as "meeting the psychosocial needs of patients." This term tends to give the impression that both the patients' needs and the workers' actions can be readily defined. Instead, this work is actually very complex and often invisible. Also, it is often made difficult because it is carried out by people who are wholly or partly strangers to the patients. Most of these care givers have only scanty information about the details of a patient's medical history, biography, and attitudes toward the illness. Although there are many ways to categorize and conceptualize this so-called psychological work, we use instead the term *sentimental work,* and distinguish subtypes: (1) trust work, (2) composure work, (3) biographical work, and (4) identity work (Strauss, Fagerhaugh, Suczek, and Wiener, 1985). These distinctions specify different conditions, consequences of carrying out each kind of work, and relationships of kinds of sentimental work to other types of trajectory work.

Sentimental work is highly complex and difficult. While the management of clinical safety is complex in and of itself, when it is combined with management of the psychological safety of the patient, then greater diligence, team communication, interactional skills, and interpersonal sensitivity are required of the staff. An important aspect of this work is that, like comfort work, it is often invisible to other staff members. Also, clinical safety predominates, so that sentimental work becomes a relatively unaccountable feature of hospital reporting. This invisibility can arouse tension among the staff, for example, when a social worker at a patient conference implies that the patient's "psychosocial needs were not met."

Sentimental work is somewhat more visible during shift changes, when staff members brief each other about the condition of patients as well as about the work done and needing to be done. Also some staff conferences focus on psychosocial problems of a specific patient. Often at these conferences, bits and pieces of biographical information that each staff member has individually learned become more generally shared, as well as the kinds of sentimental strategies that have been used. At a conference held two months after a patient's hospital admission, the chief medical resident, who just learned of her biographical history, commented, "I wish I had known about this earlier." Yet, attempts by one of the nurses to apprise him earlier were ignored or deemed irrelevant to the medical care. The physician had been occupied with clinically complex risk problems, and the nurses had been complaining about the patient's "recalcitrance." She had been seen as willfully bent on manipulating the staff. Their irritation had almost totally prevented the necessary sentimental work.

In the first sections of this chapter we shall discuss the difficulties that both the patient and staff encounter in providing relief from discomfort. First, we note the increased technologizing of discomfort, along with development of "soft technologies" to minimize discomfort, in today's hospitals. Then we examine some difficulties caused by the puzzling nature of discomfort, and we look at how this in turn poses problems in assessing discomfort, which results in strained patient-staff interactions. Notable also is the organizational context in which comfort and caring are carried out. This complex context includes care givers who have differing priorities, and these discrepancies constitute hindrances to providing discomfort relief. Then in the last part of the chapter, we shall discuss sentimental work as the second component of caring.

Discomfort Relief Technologies: Hard and Soft

In the medical arena there are now many varieties of technologies, both hard and soft, traditional and nontraditional, for relieving discomfort. In the last decade, not only has technological innovation drastically altered the nature of diagnosis and treatment, but "hard technology" has mechanized, gadgetized, and pharmacologized discomfort relief. Although these changes have made discomfort relief more effective and efficient, they have created unforeseen and sometimes undesirable, even dangerous consequences.

Evolution of the hospital bed exemplifies the mechanizing of comfort work. In the past, changing the patient's position in bed was managed manually by the nurse. Then the bed became electrified, enabling the patient to change positions merely by pushing buttons. While the mechanized bed allows a patient to do his or her own comfort work, it can result in the staff's neglect of proper body positioning. In consequence, a patient may develop still other discomfort or even have an illness course compromised. For example, a not uncommon sight in hospitals is that of patients hunched in bed, sitting on the small of their backs. This can result in backaches and even respiratory infections because of incomplete lung expansion.

Many other procedures utilized for therapeutic as well as discomfort relief—such as cold and hot applications—have become mechanized. Cool sponge baths to lower fever and relieve discomfort have been replaced by hypothermo electric machines, which are also used for heat. These and other machines come in many types and many models. "Do-it-yourself" comfort devices that were previously invented by nurses have been increasingly taken over by hospital and medical supply industries. New kinds of equipment and devices are constantly being produced and introduced—as illustrated by the briefs on new equipment published in medical and nursing journals. These new pieces of equipment and devices are extremely helpful in the sense that an electric eggbeater is certainly more efficient than a manual one. However, the innovations have called for a much more elaborate organization in order to maintain and distribute the goods and services required for comfort work.

As a result of new medical knowledge and the growth of the pharmaceutical industry, drugs are increasingly important in discomfort relief. Along with an increase in specific therapeutic drugs, a vast array of other drugs is now available for relieving such discomforts as itching, nausea, flatulence, constipation, headache, depression, and anxiety. Both medical workers and patients rely heavily on drugs for discomfort relief. Some drugs are highly effective, but since many have untoward side effects, constant upgrading of knowledge and attention are required in order to monitor the patient's physiological reaction. For a person with many discomforts, many drugs may be used. In turn, this may pose additional problems. A drug to control one discomfort may have an unfavorable effect on another discomfort, or there may be problems in identifying which of the many drugs is responsible for the appearance of a new discomfort.

In recent years there has been an increase in knowledge about the incompatibilities of drug to drug, drug to food, as well as about untoward effects of a drug for a given disease when there exists yet another disease—all matters that can affect the patient's safety (Karch and others, 1979). Nevertheless, the problem of drug incompatibility is exacerbated by the growing number of patients who have multiple chronic disorders. In large medical centers, pharmacy information centers have emerged for coping with this issue. Some centers have computerized these data. Pharmacists are becoming increasingly important in the treatment process because of the complexity of medical care when many body systems are compromised. Very specialized pharmacological knowledge is required to select appropriate drugs from among the multitude of options available today.

Besides hard technology—the machinery, various devices, and drugs—designed for discomfort relief, today's medical scene includes techniques that can be termed *soft technology*. By this we mean techniques that require much practice, skill, and art and are based on a body of knowledge drawn from both the biophysical and social sciences. Soft technology deals with appropriate ways of interacting with and taking care of the patients and their bodies so as to make patients feel physically and psychologically comfortable, be encouraged, and be assisted in managing their discomforting situations and events. Much of the "meeting of hygienic needs" and the "meeting of psychological needs" might well be conceptualized as soft technology. As nursing becomes more professionalized, the giving of discomfort relief is based more on some degree of scientific knowledge and less on common sense. Expert application of soft technology can be as effective as drugs to relieve discomfort (for instance, in allaying anxiety and depression), though both may be used.

Within the last several decades, there has been a diffusion of knowledge from the social sciences, with associated techniques for decreasing psychological and physical discomforts and distress. There are psychological approaches (both one-to-one and group), such as reflective techniques (Rogerian) and operant conditioning (Skinnerian, including biofeedback methods using machinery), along with techniques associated with various psychological schools (Jungian, Reichian, Bernian, Laingian, and so on). By and large these techniques are related to psychotherapy, but they have also influenced health professionals in their management of physically and psychologically discomforted patients.

In addition, various teaching philosophies within nursing influence discomfort work—for example, notions of self-care and dependence-independence (Bennett, 1980). Current professional ideology leads nurses to encourage the patient to move toward independence and self-care—that is, to do his or her own comfort work. However, among staff and between patient and staff there may be differing perceptions of the mode and the pacing of independence.

Another important influence beginning to affect traditional medical care is the alternative health care movement, which is partly a reaction against medical technology based on conceptions of its hazards. Alternate care groups have their own approaches to discomfort relief. Widely divergent approaches have evolved: yoga, transcendental meditation, acupuncture, herbs, folk medicine, and so on. Some of these approaches embrace varieties of exotic Eastern methods, and they range from those closely allied to traditional Western medicine to those far removed.

The foregoing discussion only partially suggests the potpourri of technologies, both hard and soft, traditional and nontraditional, now used to relieve discomfort. In the acute care hospital setting, it is safe to say that traditional (hard) technological approaches dominate. Yet the numerous approaches to discomfort relief pose the likelihood that patients and health team members will hold quite varying and potentially clashing views about appropriateness. Psychosocially oriented nurses may disapprove of colleagues who emphasize drugs as a major method of discomfort relief, since they believe drugs are clinically less effective or more hazardous. Nurses and doctors, too, of course, may disagree about appropriate drug options. Patients who ascribe to alternative health approaches may have difficulties in legitimating to staff the efficacy of divergent methods, such as the use of herbs. For example, one holistically oriented patient believed a special herb worked better than the laxative offered him. As he was an experienced patient, having had many hospitalizations for his chronic illness, rather than create a ruckus by openly refusing the laxative offered, he surreptitiously took his own herb. Also, unbeknown to the nurse, he offered his herb to roommates who gladly accepted it.

The Nature of Discomfort: Disease and Dis-ease

Pain and discomfort are usually the reasons why people seek medical help. These are interpreted as signs of illness. Logically, the focus of medical care involves discovering the cause of the pain and discomfort and then giving appropriate relief. Yet, far from being logical and orderly, relief of discomfort is highly complex work. This is readily understandable if we consider the puzzling nature of discomfort in its many varieties and examine it in an organizational and interactional context.

Discomfort can be viewed as at the less acute end of a continuum that runs from discomfort to severe pain. Discomfort is a highly subjective experience—only someone who has the discomfort perceives it. Furthermore, one person's discomfort may be defined as pain by another, or vice versa. Pain is a puzzling phenomenon, but in many ways discomfort can be more so. Discomfort can range from mundane to critical, be visible or invisible, and also may be very subtle. The ambiguities surrounding discomfort and its relief are related in part to their commonplaceness, for they are related to everyday life and to the many kinds and sources of daily discomfort that may not be related to illness. These ambiguities pose difficulties for hospitalized patients and the health workers.

Discomfort covers a wide range of physical and psychological states. Associated sensations include tingling, itching, soreness, pressure and fullness, coldness, hotness, stiffness, thirst, dirtiness. Uncomfortable physical states include weakness, dizziness, flatulence, and constipation. Discomforting psychological states and mood include "feeling blue" or "out of it," as well as unpleasant feelings derived from social situations or from interactions that result in one's feeling humiliated, ignored or slighted, embarrassed, irritated, angered, anxious, and so on. In the course of living, everybody has experienced many of the above discomforts and has developed individualized, privatized ways of managing them.

The sources of discomfort are many: they include work, social situations and interactions, as well as "normal" aging, and the physical environment itself. In addition, discomfort arises when taking care of routine bodily functions—eating, sleeping, defecating, bathing, ambulating.

In everyday life, one's own body and its discomforts tend to be a very private matter. People do not expose certain parts of their bodies in public. Caring for one's own body—housekeeping tasks such as bathing and defecating—are usually done in private. There are social norms against talking in public about intimate, "private" parts, and publicly relieving of discomfort, by passing gas, for example, or scratching oneself, is frowned upon. People often attempt to maintain a semblance of healthy bodily "normalcy." In short, everyday discomfort tends to be mundane and private. Moreover, assessments of discomfort are often based on everyday activities—an upset stomach from last night's dinner or from too much alcohol and party food; tiredness and lack of energy from too much pressure at work or family problems. In fact, even when discomfort is directly related to disease, people attempt to normalize or hide it when in social situations (Strauss and others, 1984).

This ordinary, everyday normalizing and managing of discomfort, as well as the avoidance of placing a burden on others, is drastically altered when a person is hospitalized. First of all, the medical orientation of the staff encourages the viewing of discomfort as symptomatic of disease and so of clinical danger (McBryde and Blacklow, 1970; Byers, 1975). Symptom assessment is important for proper diagnosis and treatment, and for determining the illness status, as well as for monitoring the patient's reaction to therapy. Assessments of discomfort are also important for justifying complaints about discomfort. However, because discomfort is ambiguous—stemming in part from the many possible sources that may not be directly related to disease—a patient may have the problem of deciding which particular discomforts are important enough to make public to the health workers. Over time, because of the questions asked by the latter, the patient may learn which dis-eases are significant to report or from which to request relief.

Second, emotional discomfort, such as anxiety or depression, increases in the hospital setting because new meanings are assigned to the physical discomforts. They are no longer mundane and are possibly even life-threatening. This may also encourage the patient to dwell on his or her body and its various discomforts.

Third, the previous privateness of the body becomes very public. This often results in a patient's feeling humiliated, embarrassed, or even angry. One's body comes under public scrutiny and becomes shared territory for all kinds of people who may lay claims to it. In the name of curing or at least alleviating disease, physicians, nurses, technicians, and other paraprofessionals manipulate and expose the patient's body, inserting instruments, needles, and tubes into it. The physical state of the patient's body, and sometimes even the patient's psychological state is so openly discussed among health team members that visitors and other patients may sometimes overhear the talk.

Routine bodily housekeeping tasks are done under strange conditions and with unfamiliar equipment. Sometimes minimal information is given to patients about how to go about these tasks—for instance, a basin of water may be plunked down with, "OK, get started on your bath." Some tasks are difficult, like cleaning oneself after using the bedpan, but because this is a very private matter patients ordinarily do not ask for assistance. Bodily housekeeping routines characteristically done at home are now disrupted in order that the patient may fit into hospital and ward routines.

Fourth, patients are required to cede discomfort management to others. In very acute illness states, generally patients will readily relinquish this responsibility to the staff. However, many patients suffer from chronic illnesses and, having long experience in managing their own discomfort, often have tried many types of drugs and experimented with various body positions and the pacing of activities, and so on. In many respects they may be more expert in managing their discomfort than are the personnel. Although multiple chronic illnesses are not uncommon, the staff is likely to focus primarily or solely on discomfort associated with the specific illness for which a patient has been hospitalized, to the neglect of discomfort associated with other chronic disorders.

Fifth, discomfort is also inflicted by the staff during their diagnosis and treatment of disease. A patient may have to tolerate many needle injections or irritations from tubes placed in body orifices, or maintain an uncomfortable position in order for diagnostic and treatment procedures to be successful. Today, with the increased kinds and numbers of diagnostic and treatment technologies available, there is a parallel increase in inflicted procedure-related discomfort (Fagerhaugh and Strauss,

1977). Although these technologies enable rapid diagnosing and stabilizing of the disease process, inflicted discomfort—simultaneously and serially applied—are not uncommon. Thus, when patients are admitted to the hospital, before they can become oriented to the strange environment, often they are bombarded with diagnostic procedures by various hospital workers who stream into their rooms to do various kinds of work on them. They are also being transported (with attendant discomfort) to and from specialized treatment and diagnostic sites. The medical work itself then has a potential for increasing the patient's discomfort immensely. Additionally, the patient's environment may be noisy, crowded, and untidy. The lack of privacy, the unfamiliar situation, and the loss of control of discomfort relief add to increased psychological dis-ease that in turn may affect the illness process.

Sixth, the very mundane quality of the discomfort has a peculiar effect on the health workers' perceptions of discomfort. Indeed, discomfort may be given positive meaning, as illustrated in the oft-heard phrase used by doctors and nurses when they attempt to gain a patient's cooperation for an uncomfortable treatment or procedure: "It won't be pain so much as it will be discomfort."

And a final point: the mundane character of discomfort also tends to make invisible the relief work in which both the patient and the staff engage. Patients do a great deal of relief work that may be invisible to the staff. For example, a patient may prop a pillow a certain way before a procedure is started because of a "touch of arthritis" or move in a certain way to "avoid having the back go out." The staff does not necessarily see that as the management of potentially increased discomfort. They may not even notice it. A counterpart of the invisibility of the patient's work is that the nurses' comfort work may also be invisible or misinterpreted by the patient. Nurses' comfort work often requires much skill, knowledge, technique, and art. Also, the carrying out of bodily housekeeping tasks (in nursing terms, "meeting hygienic needs" of patients) is important for its therapeutic—including safety—implications. But to a patient, this work may seem quite commonsensical or artless. A patient may merely perceive the nurse as "being nice." Nurses observe patients closely in order to assess and monitor the effects of discomfort-relieving procedures and drugs, but this work is often invisible to the patient. Hence the oft-heard criticism, "The only thing nurses do is pass out pills."

Dimensions of Discomfort

The wide variation in discomfort suffered by patients relates to the routine discomfort of everyday life as well as to the disease, the diagnostic and treatment procedures, and the particular illness phases. For each discomfort, assessments are made according to significant dimensions of the discomforts themselves. Not unlike hazard dimensions, as discussed in Chapter Two, these dimensions include duration, frequency, gravity, specificity of cause, predictability, preventability, and controllability. Duration refers to how long the discomfort lasts, and frequency refers to how often it occurs. Gravity refers to the potential seriousness of the discomfort, whether life-threatening or nonthreatening. Specificity of cause is the extent to which the origin of a discomfort can be identified. Predictability refers to the extent to which a discomfort's occurrence can be anticipated. Preventability is the extent to which it can be stopped from occurring. Controllability is the degree to which it can be held in check. Each dimension is on a continuum that will range, for instance, from high to low, short to long, ambiguous to clear-cut, and so on.

Staff take these dimensions into account when assessing discomfort and determining the related priorities of action. The degree of efficiency in discomfort relief is based on the extent to which the numbers and kinds of discomforts, and their associated dimensions, can be mapped out throughout the hospitalization. Diseases vary widely on these dimensions. For some diseases, the origins of discomfort may be obscure, but for others they may be quite clear (as for an uncomplicated appendectomy). For still others, illness control may inevitably bring inflicted pain and discomfort that are associated with the diagnostic and treatment interventions. Physicians take this discomfort into account when deciding on diagnostic and treatment options, weighing and balancing pain and discomfort against other clinical risks. Indeed, both types of risk are of much concern to physicians. Hence, the "invasiveness" and "noninvasiveness" of given diagnostic and treatment measures is a frequent point of discussion among physicians and with patients when selecting appropriate clinical options.

A central problem associated with discomfort relief is the subjectivity of pain and discomfort. This increases the chances for disagreements about discomfort priorities or dimensions not only between patient and staff but also between nurses and physicians or among nurses or physicians themselves. For instance, staff may consider a given discomfort as an indication of clinical risk and therefore give higher priority to this discomfort, but the patient may be more concerned with another discomfort (like constipation) judged by the staff as of lower priority. Or take the matter of duration of discomfort: staff may perceive the duration of a discomfort (without relief) as short, but the patient may feel its duration is interminable. Or a patient who must tolerate a discomforting treatment twice a day may think this frequency very high, but the staff may judge that the treatment needs to be increased to three times a day. Furthermore, staff may disagree among themselves about the degree of discomfort and a patient's toleration of it. Given the possibility for mismatched assessments, patients can then feel neglected or even make accusations of staff negligence. Such accusations can also occur between staff members.

Comfort Work and Other Priorities

How effectively comfort work can be accomplished depends in some part on how well it can be scheduled. Its scheduling depends on its importance relative to other work, the time available, and the degree to which the person doing the given work has control over the goods, services, and resources to do that work.

Sometimes diagnostic and treatment tasks may have higher priority than discomfort relief because of the staff's primary clinical safety focus. The increase in specialized sites within hospitals for treatment and diagnosis has increased the traffic of patients to and from specialized services. Likewise, the coming and going of various technicians and specialists to and from the patient's room has increased. The scheduling of comfort work, unless considered relevant to clinical safety, must be squeezed in between other work—not an easy job.

A related issue is that diagnostic and treatment work tends to be done during the day shift (7 A.M. to 5 P.M.), with limited services at other hours. On the day shift, attempts are made to bring order to comfort work by routinizing it—there is a time to bathe, to pass out fresh drinking water, to pass out meal trays—but the intensity of the therapeutic schedule competes with the comfort schedule. Usually the comfort scheduling loses out. Often a nurse will plan the comfort work but will not be able to carry it out because of the unexpected development of a higher-priority clinical situation—for instance, another patient suddenly hemorrhaging. In other words, the unit itself may be faced with contingencies that interrupt and throw off the comfort work schedule.

Since all departments and services have their own priorities and characteristic contingencies when work goes awry, the patients consequently may suffer unnecessary discomfort. For example, in places such as x-ray departments, the main priority is to get a good picture; the patient's discomfort is of lesser importance. Work flow there is more efficient if a batch of patients is immediately available. Thus, it is not unusual at x-ray departments to find patients queued in chairs, wheelchairs and narrow gurneys, awaiting their turn, experiencing various degrees of discomfort while doing so. In fact, a characteristic feature of this department is the discomfort associated with waiting time. A delay of schedule on these services can result in patients' comfort schedules going awry—like missing two meals in a row and so developing a hunger headache, or being thirsty for an unreasonable time because no liquids are allowed for a successful test, or experiencing a delay in receiving a drug given for discomfort relief. (Recollect, too, the case described in an earlier chapter of an elderly lady's suffering cold from waiting for a procedure and so getting a therapeutic setback.) The staff back on the nursing unit are then faced with the need to rectify the irritations and discomfort that patients develop on these specialized services, but nurses (and physicians) have little control over preventing their occurrence.

Inadequacies in goods and services from support services also greatly frustrate the work of relieving discomfort. Patients may require frequent linen changes because of excessive sweating or inability to control their bowels, or may require a comfort device or a relieving drug. Yet they may suffer because of a shortage of supplies or a wait for their next scheduled delivery. This is another instance of waiting time discomfort. It is not unusual to hear a nurse explain, ''A drug (equipment, or device) is ordered for your discomfort, but we have to wait for its delivery.'' Consequently, it is common to hear (an angry version of): ''What the hell does it take to get a pill for my headache!''

In large medical centers, support services related to discomfort relief may be insufficient because of the logistics of supply and goods, since numerous kinds of equipment and supplies must be on hand at the patient care units. To protect themselves from shortages because of the unreliable deliveries, nurses may hoard goods and equipment or demand a larger variety of stock on hand. This results in interdepartmental tensions and mutual accusations of mismanagement. One administrator who was responsible for the flow of goods throughout his hospital stated in dismay, ''I know the nurses are on the front lines and want to be prepared for all eventualities, but what they want is a medical-nursing Sears Roebuck Catalogue on Wheels!'' He added that all the hoarding prevented an accurate account of actual need of goods in order to plan a rational supply system.

A delay in machinery repair can also bring about frustration and ineffective care. For example, a delay in replacing a nonfunctioning electric bed requires that work with patients be done in a position that strains the nurse's back. This also results in work inefficiently performed at the expense of the patient's comfort.

Another set of conditions that affects the ordering of priorities is the dominant work patterns at the different work sites. For example, in intensive care units the work is organized around closely monitoring the machines and the biological systems of critically ill patients, and in applying vigorous medical interventions in order to return the body to equilibrium. Patients are often a mass of discomfort because of the numerous inflicted treatments and the monitors, which involve machines that require insertion of tubes into various parts of the body. Though ICU staff recognize comfort care as important, it may be quite secondary to bringing the body back to a state of equilibrium. Unfortunately, disruption of sleep patterns and heightened anxiety from the tense environment are by-products of the major priority of saving lives. By contrast, a cancer ward generally will have far less of an emphasis on immediate lifesaving but a great emphasis on people.

The ever expanding, complex therapeutic tasks and the associated administrative and coordination tasks therefore have resulted in delegating comfort tasks to auxiliary nursing staff. This is particularly true of routine bodily housekeeping tasks. Indeed a proponent of "touch therapy" commented that nurses touch the patient only when doing a procedure but only rarely to comfort a patient (Goodykoontz, 1979). Another consequence of delegating these comfort tasks to paraprofessionals is reducing these tasks to lesser importance than therapeutic ones, making them into "servile work" or even "dirty" work (Hughes, 1971). In addition, the nursing drive for professional and equal status among health professionals tends generally to relegate comfort work to a low status—thereby setting another, more invisible condition for increased clinical danger.

Difficulties in Discomfort Interactions

Patients have many interactional difficulties with the staff about discomfort. Because they apprise the staff about the quality and extent of their discomfort, they must convince the staff when requesting discomfort relief. They must also endure the pain if the staff thinks that is necessary, even if they themselves are unconvinced. They are supposed to express their discomfort in appropriate ways. Aside from the subtlety and subjectivity of

discomfort, which makes it very difficult for the patients to identify, they experience difficulty in identifying the staff's norms of
discomfort interactions. Quite often, unbeknown to patients,
there are implicit norms or assumptions about appropriate patient behavior associated with discomfort relief—for example,
concerning styles of requesting relief. Ordinary rules of politeness
govern how a patient should ask for relief; it is not to be done too
demandingly, nastily, or with screaming and shouting. There is
also a right time—when the nurse isn't tied up with another patient, when it does not conflict with the passing of food trays, or
within the limits of prescribed drug dose intervals (every three
hours, not every two hours). There are also norms of enduring
and tolerating discomfort and how they should be expressed. The
patient should tolerate an uncomfortable procedure because it is
necessary for getting well. Quiet moaning is acceptable but not
long, continuous, loud moaning because this upsets other patients. Indeed, the problems that patients have in figuring out the
rules of discomfort relief are great, as is evidenced by the amount
of patient-patient and patient-kin checking out and prompting.
"Don't you think you ought to ask for a pill for your_____?
Do you think I ought to tell the nurse?" or "I think you have
put up with this long enough." For the patient constantly to dwell
on bodily discomfort and express it (or its opposite, underexpressing it) may have grave interactional consequences—some
of them with safety aspects. Overreporting and overexpressing
may result in patients being labeled as hypochondriac or overanxious, while underexpressing may bring about such labels as
macho, or denier. On the other hand, the staff must manage ill
people who complain constantly, so there is also the work of
managing their own reactions to that complaining.

    Patients may also face difficulties in legitimating their
discomfort (Fagerhaugh and Strauss, 1977). Quite often the difficulties stem from differing criteria for legitimation held by staff
and patients. For the staff, legitimation is often based on technology; greater validity is placed on those discomforts that fall
within a disease's syndrome and can be objectively proven by
laboratory tests, x-rays, and so on. Conversely, the patients'
description of discomfort is sometimes not as convincing.

Balancing Within Discomfort Work: An Example

In providing comfort to the patient, a number of safety issues need to be taken into account. These include balancing the following: patient-staff interactional consequences, staff-staff interactional consequences, and patient safety–other work consequences. As an illustration, take a simple comfort task—giving a bed bath on the second postoperative day after a hysterectomy. In commonsense terms, the bath is meant to refresh and make the patient more comfortable. Should the registered nurse or the aide do the work? Or should the patient be encouraged to do her own comfort work? To a professional nurse, the bed bath is more than a commonsense comfort procedure; it is a vehicle to observe the patient and her bodily signs. Where possible, the patient is encouraged to give her own bath as this activity helps her maintain muscle tone and stimulates circulation and respiration, which in turn may prevent complications. Also, the activity will help to move the patient toward greater "independence," meaning less work for the personnel and also sometimes speeded up recovery. In other words, this work must be balanced against and in tandem with the patient's safety.

Should the nurse decide to balance on the side of encouraging the patient to do her own comfort work, then the nurse must persuade her so as to avoid the consequences of being accused of being hardhearted and unsympathetic—an attack on the nurse's personal and professional identity. A great deal of personal presence and appropriate persuasion may be required, especially when the patient reacts with, "It's only my second day after surgery, and I'm weak," or "At $200 a day I have to take my own bath!" As noted earlier, within the nursing staff there may be varying notions of pacing toward independence. One nurse may judge the patient as too sick to do her own work and feel it is hazardous to have her attempt it; another may judge that the emotional state of the patient is such that she needs the touch contact. Still another may judge this as babying the patient, while another believes that the therapeutic aspects of independence are of importance here.

If the nurse opts to do comfort work for the patient, while the head nurse or the team leader is oriented toward pushing the patient toward independence (and perhaps also is more concerned with the unit's overall treatment work requirements), then the nurse's decision may be criticized. This is yet another contingency that brings about a bruised personal and professional identity. Again, a nurse may balance comfort work against other ongoing work and may decide to assign the task to an aide. The aide may have different notions of dependence-independence or see the work only in commonsensical terms. On the other hand, the aide may feel burdened with dirty work.

Nurses and Comfort Care

Among the health professionals, it is generally accepted that comfort safety is in the nurses' domain, but the increase in immediate medical/technical hazard concerns has prevented their closer attention to discomfort work. Over the years, as professional nurses have relinquished much routine body comfort work to other personnel—such as licensed vocational nurses and nurse's aides—they have also lost control over organizational resources to do this and other work. As discussed in the chapter on major safety work processes (Chapter Four), the intricate overlapping of comfort, clinical, identity, and interactional safety poses problems for nurses in their management of discomfort hazards. Also, where the discomforts are clinically derived or related, rectifying may call for delicate negotiations or even outright confrontations with many other types and levels of workers. Then, too, because nurses are on the front lines of care, they are recipients of the reactions of disgruntled and angry patients, even though the source of the patients' discomfort may be their mismanaged care by other workers.

Ironically, the professionalization of nursing has itself posed difficulties in doing comfort work. This work, legitimated by an underpinning of science and scientific principles, has been redefined as "therapeutic" intervention. It is interesting to note the growing interest in "touch therapy." The use of touch to comfort the patient is now legitimized by an extensive conceptual framework (Goodykoontz, 1979; Weiss, 1979). Such technologizing of comfort care seems necessary today in order for that work to be rendered more legitimate. A paradoxical situation develops—comforting for its own humane sake is not necessarily legitimate, but must be therapeutic and based as much as possible on scientific principles. Implicit here is the assumption, too, that care then will be not only more effective but also safer.

Sentimental Work

Moral Rules of Interaction. Before discussing these subtypes, we should note that there are some implicit understandings (taken-for-granted norms or rules) that underlie interaction. In order to avoid arousing feelings of depersonalization in others, people must follow these implicit norms or rules: that is, each must regard others as considerate, reasonable, and polite (Garfinkel, 1967). Thus, between interactants there exist implicit contracts. In conversations one is expected to listen attentively, make appropriate gestures (such as nodding), not break in abruptly, not shout, to be pleasant and tactful when making requests of others, and follow the social norms that govern privacy and intimacy (Goffman, 1963). A person who breaks these implicit norms is regarded as inconsiderate, discourteous, and rude, while the others may feel humiliated, deprecated, and depersonalized because of the improper behavior.

When strangers meet, there are implicit rules in effect, such as the necessity of introducing oneself and showing appropriate respect to persons of different status. Hence, when a young nurse addressed an elderly patient by his given name, he icily responded, "I am Mr. Smith to you, not John." Or a doctor who began to ask a woman patient many questions without first introducing himself was asked, "Who are you?" To his reply, "I'm your anesthesiologist," her response was, "Not if I have anything to say about it!"

Aside from everyday interactional rules, there are some that pertain particularly to body work. Thus, workers who handle patients' bodies must first obtain their consent. Permission may often be indirect—some explanation as to why the work is necessary. At the same time, patients should be told what the work will entail, their associated tasks, the unpleasant aspects of the work, and how those aspects will be controlled.

A second rule, as mentioned earlier, is that privacy is protected as much as possible in order to minimize embarrassment. Frequently, when there is an intense medical focus (particularly when patients are in very risky physical states that require immediate access to the body), then adherence to this implicit rule may be neglected. At such places as the intensive care units, exposed bodies and lack of privacy are usual. It is a common situation in large teaching hospitals—where patients' privacy is often invaded and so feelings of depersonalization are generated— that patients are used as "teaching cases." Especially demeaning to patients are examinations done or procedures performed in the presence of students and residents on the genital, rectal, or breast areas. For example, one female patient had a vaginal procedure performed in the presence of four medical students; so intent was the senior physician in his teaching, and the medical students in learning, that little explanation and attention was paid to the patient. After the physicians left the room, she broke out in sobs because of her humiliation.

A third implicit interactional rule is that when handling the body, the worker should minimize inflicted pain and discomfort. And when unavoidable, the patients must be apprised of the pain or discomfort they must endure (Fagerhaugh and Strauss, 1977).

All of these body work rules have the instrumental value of getting work done efficiently, but they also decrease patients' anxieties and assist them in maintaining composure. When the rules are broken—because of workers' insensitivity, conditions such as teaching taking precedence over patient comfort, or emergency situations—patients may define workers in negative terms, and trust may deteriorate. Of course, this can very much increase the chances of hazards in their care.

Trust Building. To gain patients' cooperation for efficiently accomplishing necessary work requires gaining and maintaining trust. Gaining trust involves much time, talk, sensitivity, and demonstration of competence. Patients must perceive staff members as genuinely and sincerely interested in their well-being and welfare, possessing honesty and openness in dealing with patients, and being clinically competent. The building of trust rests in part on adherence to various implicit interactional rules. Breaking them can shatter trust or at least make the building of trust very difficult.

Building trust also requires a high degree of sensitivity to patients' moods and reactions. Unless patients are skillfully invited to express their fear, anxieties, and disgruntlement about the care, the staff members may experience difficulty in the kinds of interactions necessary for establishing or reestablishing trust. In fact, the trust work called for will vary widely by phases of a trajectory, the kinds and quality (risk, pain, patient participation, and so on) of the tasks, as well as patients' moods and biographies. Generally, if the task to be performed is simple and routine, involving minimal risk, then a polite and pleasant interaction and a show of competence will suffice.

Since much care revolves around the managing of hazards, trust work involves apprising patients about hazards, while at the same time demonstrating competence in their management. This is done not only by possessing technical competence and judgment but also by evincing calmness, steadiness, and self-confidence. Of course, apprising patients of potential risks has recently gained in emphasis as a result of the patients' rights movement and the subsequent use of informed consent, along with concern over the legal consequences of not informing patients. Under conditions of great clinical risk where the clinical outcomes may be highly problematic, trust work is rendered extremely difficult, particularly for phsicians who are largely responsible for this work in those conditions. As discussed earlier, risk disclosure by physicians is extremely difficult. Physicians must disclose without overly frightening their patients, as well as make decisions about pacing their disclosures. In this regard, risk disclosure may be seen as a variety of awareness context work (Glaser and Strauss, 1965): that is, sentimental effort by the staff either to disclose or withhold information in order to protect or maintain patients' identities or maintain their composures.

Trust work occurs within the context of busy, fast-moving wards where many workers interact with each patient. Uncontrolled and invisible events can decrease trust between them.

In the following episode, one can see varied events and conditions that contribute to a breakdown in trust.

> A middle-aged male who was having chronic, painful hemifacial spasms was referred to a medical neurologist at a reputable university hospital. After examining him, the neurologist referred this patient to a neurosurgeon at the same hospital. The latter explored the possibility of doing a very special type of surgical procedure. It has many potential risks, among them an unavoidable permanent deafness. The patient fully expected that the neurosurgeon could be trusted since he was told that the surgeon was extremely competent and that the surgical technique had been developed at this same hospital. The surgeon was young and very busy, not only with his own practice but also with research and with training house staff and medical students. He relied heavily on the staff for most of the initial physical examination and explanations of the care given to the patient.
>
> During the early phases of hospitalization, this "case" was discussed at house staff rounds led by the chief resident, but with the neurosurgeon absent. At this time the patient remarked to one of us that since entering the hospital, he had been having fewer facial spasms. During the rounds an intern asked the patient why he would consider undergoing a potentially risky surgery "just for cosmetic purposes." The physicians were entirely unaware of the long years that the patient had had of painful facial spasms and how it had affected his life. For instance, his eating and talking or sudden changes in temperature (as when going outside) would often trigger painful spasms. Increasing pain and spasms had greatly interfered with his social interactions. The lack of biographical information about him was due in part to the physician's focus

on taking a medical history. The patient felt humiliated and angry, for the remark "just for cosmetic
purposes" indicated that his pain was not legitimate
and that he was a vain man. When asked the question about why have the surgery in the presence
of several house staff but with no physician there
to mitigate or at least assuage him about the unsympathetic remark, he felt very vulnerable. It took
great effort to control his desire to tell the questioner
off—"Who are you to tell me if I have or don't have
pain!" When the resident discussed the surgical
risks, he did it with little finesse—in fact, the patient described it as "brutal."

Meanwhile, the attending neurosurgeon,
though pleasant, gave out an air of being busy. The
patient was visited by him either in the context of
teaching rounds or after having attended two acutely
ill roommates of the patient. Several house staff informed the patient that the surgeon was highly competent and had much experience with this particular
surgical technique. Because the very sick roommates required much care, this patient felt reluctant to impose on the staff. Most interactions by
the nurses with him were in regard to various diagnostic tests. Desperate for pain relief, he made the
hard decision to go ahead with the surgery. He was
scheduled for it at a future date.

Then his medically sophisticated sister sensed
that all was not well, basing her judgment partly
on the surgeon's unavailability, the interactional
ineptness of the chief resident, and the unspoken
uneasiness expressed by her brother. When she
asked him if he had doubts about the neurosurgeon
and whether the services of another might be explored, he was immensely relieved. This was followed by a long list of complaints, among them was
being treated like a guinea pig by "pip-squeak"
house staff who had no "bedside manners." Intense

anger at having to justify his facial pain was also expressed. Although he did not doubt the technical competence of the neurosurgeon, he did not trust the house staff on whom he heavily relied.

His sister searched for another surgeon; this one was replaced by an older neurosurgeon who had actually pioneered the surgical technique. She advised her brother that although a good bedside manner is important, still given the high surgical risks the main emphasis was clinical competence and a surgeon who could command control over the medical care given by his assistants.

Of course, the neurosurgeon was forewarned that he needed to establish patient trust. The physician spent the first portion of the initial interview gathering biographical information: how the illness interfered with the patient's life, the kinds of treatment tried by the various physicians and their effects, the varieties of nonmedical means used to control and minimize the painful spasms, and how the patient managed social interactions. The patient commented on the calm and unhurried manner of the doctor when surgical risks were being discussed—a great contrast to the preceding physician. This one's unhurried and confident air, plus the deference shown him by house staff and nursing staff, all served to increase trust.

This case illustrates several things: (1) how structural conditions (such as a busy work schedule due to the presence of very sick patients and competing demands of teaching and learning work) can interfere with the availability of time that is necessary to build trust; (2) how the failure to do biographical work contributed to the resident's inappropriate remark; and (3) how in the taking of medical histories, appropriate pacing and ordering of the information gathering can affect the patient's building of trust in a physician. Moreover, although the house staff had attempted to build trust in the technical competence

of their superior, their efforts were countervailed by their interactional insensitivities and harmed by their superior's continuing unavailability to the patient. Further, the family-staff interactions can affect the patient's trust. As seen in this instance
both the patient and his sister grew to distrust the first surgeon.
It is usual for patients and their family members to develop different degrees of trust in a physician or to base their trust on
differing criteria. In fact, when the staff has successfully established trust with family members, then the latter may engage
in trust work with the patient on behalf of the staff.

Patients know implicitly they must behave in such a manner that they are seen as cooperative and trusting. Recognizing that they possess little medical technical knowledge, they
generally want to trust the staff. However, their growing awareness of mistakes made in medical care by health workers—fanned
in part by media reports on mismanaged care plus their own
or family's or friends' experiences with either mismanagement
or dehumanized care—makes trust work by the staff extremely
difficult. For instance, a woman undergoing therapy for breast
cancer, who had had several bad experiences in medical care,
thoroughly grilled her physicians about the various therapies
and the risk options as well as about the reliability of their creden-
tials, before accepting either the type of therapy suggested or
the particular person who would carry out the treatment.

The building and reestablishing of trust—necessary for
maximizing clinical safety—must continue throughout the entire trajectory. Informing patients about their progress, or why
it has been delayed, through the use of appropriate phrases and
gestures, serves to build trust. Hence, complaints by patients
and families that "nobody tells me anything" or "I don't know
what's going on" can be regarded as reflecting inadequate trust
work. There are certain trajectory moments when trust work
is crucial: when patients express disgruntlement about their care,
when the illness trajectory goes off course, or when patient or
family perceive the recovery is unduly delayed.

Composure Work. As frequently mentioned in these pages,
many procedures expose patients to a potential loss of composure
(poise, "face," self-control). Much of this work is carried out

by explaining and orienting patients to the work that needs to
be done. Holding hands, touching the brow, or uttering encouraging phrases like "hang in there; it will soon be over"
serve to assist patients through frightening procedures and lessen
the risks of those procedures. Indeed, procedure-related composure work is probably the most visible type of sentimental
work in the hospital. Composure work is especially important
when patients and families are given information that is difficult
for them to handle, such as the probability of continued physical
deterioration or of death.

As noted earlier, staff also engage in composure work with
themselves, in handling dirty work, in coping with their feelings of helplessness when caring for patients who continue to
deteriorate, and in managing particularly difficult patient-staff
interactions. Frequently, staff-staff composure work can be
observed, as when many deaths occur one after the other on
the unit.

Biographical Work. Biographical work is a type of work
that takes into account the patient's life history and life-style.
It is done routinely whenever physicians seek information about
patients' "social history" as this may pertain to their symptoms
and diseases. Nurses also routinely gather biographical information as part of the hospital admission process. Since they
are largely responsible for body comfort work, much of the
biographical information that they seek relates to food allergies, sleep and bowel patterns, and the like. More often than
not, this information is gathered in a matter-of-fact manner
and through rapid-fire questioning. Ordinarily, a minimum
of biographical information is gotten for carrying out the clinical work, but it can be quite important. This becomes apparent
when gravely ill patients are admitted to the hospital and are
unable to give either medical or personal information and have
no family or friends to supply the information. Then diagnosis is made more difficult. Even if the patient is conscious
or not gravely ill, biographical information—along with other
life-style cues (language, dress, and so on)—are necessary for
guiding the interactional style used by staff to elicit medical
information.

Although there is general recognition that biographical information is important and patient interview schedules identify the kinds of information to gather, the immediacy of clinical work may interfere with the amassing of information. Instances when biographical work is done purposefully include when the therapy is prolonged (as in chemotherapy for cancer) and when patients or families must participate in portions of the posthospital medical care (as with home dialysis). Information about patients' patterns of living, relationships with families, disruptions of family relationships that result from the therapy or disability, and so on are crucial for adapting the medical and nursing care to these life-styles and social situations.

Biographical information is nowadays becoming increasingly important because patients with chronic illness predominate in our hospitals. Prolonged illness and its therapy affect the biographies and life-styles in individually unique ways. When biographical information work is neglected, then the trajectory may be negatively affected: for instance, in the selection of inappropriate treatment options, resistance of patients to therapy, mispacing in the exchange of information, and unwittingly wounded sensibilities.

Identity Work. Identity work is closely related to biographical work but is analytically distinct. While biographical work pertains mainly to the obtaining of personal information, identity work refers to work done with patients that deals with matters of retaining personal identity. It is most often referred to by staff as handling "psychosocial problems." This latter type of work is concerned with helping patients to maintain their sense of personal identity, since it may be threatened or damaged by prolonged and difficult illness. This work is especially important when the disease or the medical intervention is very disabling, disfiguring, or stigmatizing. It includes helping patients to face the realities of their physical conditions and preparing them for their posthospital lives. But, of course, it is also relevant to their behavior and decisions that, in turn, increase or decrease the hazards of their illness and clinical care.

Summary

A major staff responsibility is to manage physical and psychological discomfort that often accompanies illness and its treatment. Two components of the work of caring are comfort work and sentimental work. Both are complex types of work, and are rendered even more so by constantly evolving medical technologies. Both types are embedded in the total clinical work, since in doing any intervention ''on'' the patient, inflicted discomfort and psychological dis-ease associated with the intervention should be managed. Comfort and sentimental work are essential for clinical safety.

To summarize some of what has been discussed previously about comfort work: in the first place, much uncertainty is associated with the phenomena of pain and discomfort—with their sources and their assessments. Second, the intensity of the clinical safety work competes with comfort work, for the former generally has higher priority. Third, patients are important participants in comfort work, but the patients have problems in doing their work effectively. All of this can bring about staff agreements and disagreements over aspects of comfort work, as well as interactional difficulties between staff and patients that can affect comfort care and clinical safety itself. Some changes in nurses' philosophies and actions with regard to comfort care were explored. We also discussed the consequences of competition between medical-nursing work and the minimizing of discomfort, and the conditions affecting the mitigation of this competition. Running through all of this discussion as a persistent theme was the great impact of contemporary medical technology, both ''hard'' and ''soft,'' on the changing character of comfort work.

In the second part of the chapter, some complexities of sentimental work were explored with regard to clinical safety. Several subtypes of sentimental work were distinguished, including trust work, composure work, biographical work, and identity work. We also noted a few implicit moral rules affecting interaction that pertain to sentimental work. Like comfort

work, sentimental work is often invisible to other staff members.
On medical charts, there are countless recorded details of the
technical medical work but a paucity of references to sentimental work.

Visible or invisible, accountable or not accountable, sentimental work and comfort work go on throughout the entire
trajectory. The clinical aims per phase and their associated safety
aspects ideally call for safety work that incorporates those caring aspects. Whether the caring work is done effectively, appropriately, or even at all, depends very much on organizational
conditions and arrangements.

8

Coordinating the Safety Work
of Hospital Staff

The safe management of a trajectory ultimately rests on the articulation (fitting together) both of work processes and the important types of safety work. The extent to which they can be articulated depends on how well the various hazards associated with trajectory phases can be anticipated and mapped out. Safety articulation is an effort to rationalize (make explicit the division of labor) and coordinate work in order to achieve maximum clinical safety.

Safety articulation is not, however, simply another type of work. It is much more useful to conceptualize it as another work process that enters into the entire course of a trajectory. Indeed, articulation is so central to clinical safety (as well as to other organization goals like efficiency, cost, and humaneness of care) that we can think of it as a suprawork process. Analytically speaking, it stands above the principal processes of monitoring, assessing, preventing, and rectifying. The articulation process is so central because despite these supportive processes and the hospital/ward structures, there still are those numerous contingencies, detailed in foregoing chapters, that lead to the disarticulation of safety work. There also is the obvious necessity of achieving its effective rearticulation. Ultimately this suprawork process is by far the least well understood, pragmatically and analytically.

These considerations lead us to note that there are at least four major issues attending the articulation process: 1) the difficulties in rationalizing safety work, 2) the difficulties in attaining its effective coordination, 3) the sources of its disarticulation, and 4) how articulation is achieved in spite of the numerous disarticulations. Our discussion of these issues is likely to dishearten readers at first, because of our enumeration of the very many sources of potential hazard and the consequent disarticulation of safety work. Yet there are also conditions that foster the articulation and rearticulation of this work, leading to the relative assurance that hospitals are not *that* dangerous. In this chapter, we detail both sides of this equation.

Rationalization of Medical Work

As hospitals become increasingly complex and as health care costs rise, industrial work management models are adopted to bring greater efficiency of work through the rationalization of work processes. In the last several decades, business language has pervaded health care; for instance, there is the "health industry," patients are "products," and patient care is the "production process." Certainly, some features of industrial production work can be applied to hospitals for achieving more efficient and rational work alignment and processes. In contrast, if medical production work is seen primarily as trajectory safety work, then the rational industrial work model falls far short.

In that model, the product—an automobile, for example—involves the application of scientific discoveries and engineering principles during the experimental phase, at which time a number of options are weighed and put on trial, and as far as possible the "bugs" are eliminated. The articulation of necessary resources and the meshing of thousands of tasks involved in the production process are planned beforehand. Unexpected contingencies that can interrupt the production process are anticipated as much as possible. Only then does production begin.

Effective articulation of industrial work rests on sets of conditions that foster rationalization of the production process. These include the following: (1) products are uniform and of limited numbers of models, (2) goals are clear-cut and unambiguous, (3) task components of the production are known, predictable, and unambiguous, (4) decision making is minimal, being guided by the goals, and (5) evaluation of work processes are regulated and unambiguous (Gerson, 1977).

When medical/health production is compared to industrial production, rationalizing and articulating appear to be extremely difficult. To use an analogy, a hospital is like an automobile maintenance and repair shop, but the numbers and types of its damaged products are more diverse. Of course, for greater work efficiency the hospital attempts to rationalize its work by grouping the products into similar types or degrees of damage, or according to the types of repair work to be done. However, despite the ability to do temporary repair and maintenance work, the outcomes are highly problematic and unpredictable. This is particularly the case as a damaged product ages and multiple parts become even more damaged. Moreover, although the products may be grouped according to similar types of damage, they are often in different phases of damage or phases of repair—and this makes a uniform, programmed, assembly line task approach extremely difficult. A central difference, also, is that the products (patients) are not inanimate objects. They themselves are integral to the production process and may be a source of disarticulation. Frequently, the work procedures are still being researched, as when new kinds of repair technologies are being developed or used. Thus, the means are still in the process of exploration and are subject to change. For all these reasons, the work processes in hospitals are likely to be frequently disrupted and require continual decision making to handle the disruptions. All of this results in problems of evaluation, involving criteria often yet to be created.

Sources of Disarticulation

The difficulties encountered in rationalizing and articulating safety work are imbedded within the nature of hazards in medical/health work—frequently unpredictable and problematic, and at the same time requiring much overlapping of work among many types and levels of workers who attempt to control and manage the hazards. Of course, this has already been discussed in detail, but it is summarized here with regard to the articulation of safety work.

First, dangers and risks can come from multiple sources: from the patient's disrupted physical body system and the patient's behavior, from the varieties of clinical intervention by the personnel, and the environment. These sources are highly interactive, for an increased hazard from one source can affect others. Knowledge of how these sources interact determines the criteria used to establish danger/safety limits and becomes the basis for the kinds of work processes (assessing, monitoring, and so on) engaged in by the various workers, throughout the various trajectory phases. Difficulties are encountered in rationalizing and articulating these when the hazard source interactions are unpredictable and uncertain because of limited knowledge, when the intervention applied is still very new, when multiple body systems are disrupted or the disruptions are very advanced, and/or when multiple kinds of clinical interventions are applied. Of course, efforts are made to rationalize the work processes whenever the hazard source interaction is known and anticipated. However, the hospital scene today is characterized by large numbers of patients whose illness trajectories are highly unstable for reasons cited earlier (Chapter Two). Of course, efforts are made to rationalize some aspects of safety work: safety engineers attempt to manage and control environmental hazards, various technicians attempt to manage hazards arising from machinery, and "risk managers" attempt to control external-internal hospital risk pertaining to legal or regulatory agencies. However, other personnel (and patients, too) whose main responsibility is neither environmental nor the safety of machines must of necessity share in this safety work.

Because the sources of hazards are interactive, the work processes are inextricably linked. Thus, a misassessing of hazards can lead to mismonitoring, mispresenting, and misrectifying. One of these processes may dominate during different trajectory phases, but others are almost always integral to the total safety work. Efforts to rationalize this work are made through designating certain types and levels of workers to be accountable for certain kinds or degrees of hazards during different phases and miniphases of the trajectory. Since the work processes overlap, great effort to articulate them is necessary. This is especially so when assessing and monitoring is managed by one level of worker, but rectifying can only be done by another level. Furthermore, this articulation is contingent upon agreements over the criteria of hazard/safety limits and the work involved for all parties to the work. Disarticulation of work processes can occur when the criteria of the limits are uncertain or when staff disagree about these criteria.

The work processes pertain to managing several lines of patient safety work, which include the clinical, identity, biographical, body comfort, and patient-staff interactional work. These lines of safety work apply both at the trajectory and task level. Characteristically, one or more may dominate at certain phases or miniphases of the trajectory, but the other lines are almost always linked. This is especially true for clinical safety. For instance, although clinical safety issues dominate in carrying out technical medical/nursing tasks, all the other lines of work are important components of the minitasks of an overall clinical task. All of these must be assessed, monitored, prevented, and rectified, and also simultaneously and sequentially ordered along with the clinical task. For instance, if patient identity, composure, and comfort minitasks are omitted, poorly managed, or improperly synchronized, then the primary clinical task may be discombobulated. A botched-up clinical task may affect the overall trajectory; it may also lower a patient's trust in the staff, thereby disrupting the patient-staff interactional safety so necessary for clinical safety.

In sum, the combination of multiple interrelated work processes, in relation to the several interrelated lines of safety work, calls for the articulation of many kinds and levels of workers, much of whose work overlaps. When all of these factors are combined with the many kinds of hazard sources—whose interaction may be unknown, uncertain, or unpredictable—then considerable difficulties are encountered in rationalizing safety work. Hence, there is great potential for disarticulation. Disruptions of one work process or one line of safety work, within the trajectory or task level, can disarticulate other processes and lines of safety work. That is, task-level disruptions can disrupt trajectory-level work; likewise, disruptions at the trajectory level can affect task-level work.

To illustrate this complex interaction, we shall discuss the preventing and handling of respiratory infections that patients undergoing certain types of surgery are very likely to develop unless these are carefully "managed." (We have purposely chosen a very routine example.) During the preoperative phase, prevention of potential respiratory infections—among many other potential risks—is a major responsibility of the attending nurses. This risk-prevention work is recognized by other personnel as directly within the nurses' province. This work involves helping and encouraging patients to cough up phlegm and to take deep breaths at periodic intervals. Sometimes a simple inspirator gadget may be used to facilitate deep breathing. These tasks are relatively simple and straightforward. Indeed, much of this preventive work can be done by patients.

So, what is there to articulate in these uncomplicated tasks? Although the work is simple, patients often find it difficult because the taking of deep breaths, particularly when combined with the coughing up of phlegm—and most of all when abdominal or chest surgery has been done—can be quite painful during the postoperative period. To carry out the preventive tasks, it is necessary for nurses to coordinate those with the comfort tasks: that is, to schedule the former at a time when the postoperative pain is not at its peak. Since the patient's cooperation will be essential, it is necessary during the preoperative phase for the nurses to carry out a set of information tasks concerning the potential risk of respiratory infection. Patients are informed that although the preventive tasks done later may add to their discomfort, nevertheless it is extremely important to carry them out. They are also taught how to do these tasks and the measures to be taken later for the control of pain. The staff generally believe that the preoperative rather than the postoperative phase is the more appropriate time to give this information, since directly after the operation the patients are often unable to absorb the information because of heavy medication. In the process of preventing respiratory infections, a nurse must assess the patient's potential for developing respiratory infections; the criteria will include age, types of surgery, and general cardiovascular status. These assessments will determine how frequently and vigorously the preventive tasks are carried out. Also involved is the monitoring of specific signs and symptoms for determining if the current preventive tasks need to be altered.

Compared with safety-work articulation done during the preoperative phase of surgery, this work is not considered especially complicated. However, the safety work in this postoperative phase can be readily disrupted. Why? First of all, diverse kinds of uncontrolled contingencies may disrupt the work order, not only then but all along the future course of the trajectory. Quite often the exchange of information with a patient is omitted, for various reasons: the nurse forgot this responsibility under the pressure of other tasks, the surgery was of an emergency variety so there was little time for doing those information tasks, or the patients were not mentally alert because of their illnesses. Consequently, this omission of tasks may result in great resistance later by patients to doing the coughing and deep breathing, especially because it can be so discomforting. Second, this preventive work is linked with comfort work, especially that of dealing with pain. Thus, disruption in pain assessment, monitoring, or prevention can disarticulate the clinical safety tasks. Unexpected pain-medication allergies can also occur, including nausea and vomiting. Those can disrupt fluid and electrolyte balances if continued for long periods, which thus then requires assessment, monitoring, prevention, and, if necessary, rectification work. In addition, the physician's assessment of pain may be off the mark, and therefore the prescribed medication may not control the pain.

In other words, the management of comfort and safety work here involves two or three overlapping levels of work— the physician's (or physicians'), the nurses' (several of them), and probably the patient's, too. Rectifying and rearticulating the comfort work will require exchange of information among all three levels. If the patient cannot be persuaded to do the risk prevention tasks and also has a past medical history indicating predisposition to respiratory infections, then both medication and respiratory machinery may be resorted to for loosening phlegm and facilitating deep breathing. This later work makes necessary the attendance of a respiratory therapist, whose tasks must then be articulated with all the others. But the nurses' pain tasks perhaps may not be well synchronized with the therapist's clinical tasks because the therapist was delayed by another patient who was located on another unit. Still other types of rearticulation are called for by a machine failure. And if the patient does indeed develop a respiratory infection, then the physicians must reassess and alter the trajectory scheme. That, again, affects the alignment of safety work done at the task level. Furthermore, a patient may develop distrust in the staff, so that this calls for correcting the damaged interaction between patient and staff. There is thus a constant ebb and flow of disrupted safety work. Consequently, safety priorities are constantly shifting.

For any given group of patients, when a realignment of work for a given patient is required, this will bring out a realignment of work done for other patients in that group. Effective articulation then rests on being able to anticipate how various work processes and lines of safety work interact over time. Recollect that usually safety work is organized around the phases of appearance of a hazard: (1) preventing, (2) might go wrong, (3) definitely going wrong, and (4) out of hand. During each of these phases and with each degree of hazard, the kinds of safety tasks will vary. More often than not, as degree of hazard increases, then a larger number of different kinds and levels of workers are involved. In consequence, the chances for disarticulation of safety work will increase. To make matters still more complicated, recollect that the staff can vary widely in how they assess danger and risks, and in how they balance them. Also remember that new technologies are constantly being introduced, which makes the articulation of safety work additionally contingent. In accordance with the changing technology, new workers may be introduced; and, of course, it takes time to determine where their tasks overlap with those of traditional workers, what are the limits of their task jurisdiction, and so on. All in all, safety articulation presents to the personnel and patient— and to us as researchers also—an immensely complicated picture.

The articulation must bring into alignment the several work processes and the several lines of safety work for three levels of work: (1) the overall arc of work, (2) the managerial and organizational work, and (3) the implicated tasks. Within each level, as well as among the levels, there is articulation work to be done. The physician will have a picture of both the overall safety work required and the order of tasks needed to keep the trajectory on track. He/she will articulate that part of the work that is related to his or her trajectory responsibilities. However, a large part of the organizing and managing of articulation work is done by middle-level administrators, quite often the head nurse or supervisors: for instance, the articulation of work with that of other hospital departments, along with the supervision of nurses and other personnel. Finally, there is the articulation of bundles of tasks at the task level. Disarticulations can frequently occur because so much safety work involves the alignment of workers who come from other hospital departments that may face unanticipated contingencies, and these may disarticulate the ward's work.

The staff themselves have safety concerns about their own staff-staff interactions, identities, and composures. Hence, their concerns may override that of the patient's safety. Moreover, the central hospital administrators enter into such issues as the allocation of resources for assuring safety, the safety work jurisdiction of workers, and the establishment of organizational arrangements and their articulation done to facilitate safety work. Disarticulation of safety work can occur when misassessments are made about the safety requirements believed necessary for allocating resources at the unit level or when there is inadequate articulating of organizational arrangements or mispreventing and mismonitoring of safety rules and safety needs.

An especially paradoxical feature of safety work is that its rationalization can actually lead to disarticulation! For instance, in order to assure more efficient use of resources and clinical safety, increasingly the care units are organized around homogeneous groups: according to types of illness, types of interventions, or degrees of hazard. This strategy has certainly improved the articulation of safety work within the homogeneous groups. However, during the trajectory course patients are moved from one speciality workshop to another, and thus disarticulation can occur in the transfer process. Vital information may not be transmitted. Moreover, it is not always possible to have an entirely homogeneous group of patients. Because of a shortage of hospital beds, an abdominal surgery patient may be placed in a neurosurgical unit. While the articulation work may be hampered by nurses' unfamiliarity with this patient's physician, they may also be unfamiliar with the kinds of articulation work required when caring for this kind of patient. Or patients still in potentially hazardous states may be moved out of a cardiac intensive care unit to an intermediate care unit, in order to accommodate the influx of more seriously ill patients, but the intermediate unit may be unprepared for that degree of hazard in a patient's condition. In other words, there are many conditions when patients do not "fit" the rationalized work routines for specialized patients; hence, work becomes disarticulated.

Then, of course, sources outside the hospital may disarticulate safety work, too. Clinical safety depends in part on the companies that produce the medical technologies. Defective products, inadequate arrangements for maintenance and repair, or unsatisfactory arrangements for procuring parts will disrupt safety work. Furthermore, legislation that pertains to increases or decreases in financial assistance to patients, health professionals, or health services, as well as regulatory legislation that pertains to the production of medical devices or health care practices, can enhance or disrupt trajectory safety work.

Currently, safety work and its articulation have been profoundly altered by the 1983 enactment of DRG (Diagnostic Related Group) legislation, passed in order to contain hospital costs. Although our substantive comments on it may soon be outdated, we shall discuss this legislation as an instance of how external regulation can greatly disarticulate aspects of the safety (and other) work within hospitals, and between them and other facilities, and so necessitate considerable (probably costly) efforts at rearticulation. However, the enactment of DRG has increased some hazards, but it has helped to articulate some aspects of safety work.

Under this legislation, an attempt is made to contain costs by rationing and limiting the length of hospitalization and treatment options prior to hospitalization. This is based on diagnosis and acuity of the various illnesses. Without here going into the details of how diagnosis and acuity are determined, suffice to say that this approach attempts to rationalize costs by grouping patients according to diagnostic groups, with defined norms for treatment and numbers of allowable hospital days. Based on these diagnostic groups and norms for treatment, appropriate accounting forms have been developed to control and monitor costs.

According to Robert Fetter (Fetter and others, 1980), one of the authors of the DRG legislation, the cost concern is focused on the completed course of treatment. Additionally, the quality of care is presumed stable, and the monitoring and controlling of cost does not attempt to measure the degree of care accomplished during the hospitalization or the state of the patients' health at discharge. In other words, the work or its quality (safety being one important component of quality) is not considered. The legislation is primarily concerned with cost of medical production before and after hospitalization, rather than with the quality of care. The reason is that quality of care is determined by PSRO (Professional Standards Review Organization) and the peer review process.

Hospitals have engaged in major work reorganization to meet these cost limitations. Their rearrangements include rationalizing the work, for several possible reasons: to complete more efficiently the necessary treatment work within the legislatively allowable days of hospitalization, to shift the pretreatment work (such as diagnostic tests) previously done in the hospital but now to be done at the physicians' offices or in the outpatient departments, or to increase the number of "come and go" treatments (treatments where the patient is admitted in the morning and discharged the same day). Thus, there is now a visible increase in requisite articulation work between doctors' offices and outpatient departments in relation to the inpatient services. Since organizational arrangements and the articulation of services are still in the process of development, a number of unanticipated disruptions are, of course, usual. As one nurse remarked, "We're only on the second week of this change (doing a major portion of the preliminary work for a heart catheterization in the clinic), so we are having lots of problems working out the connection with the inpatient department. It will take a couple more weeks to work it all out."

Since the enactment of the DRG legislation, both its negative and positive consequences are becoming evident. The economic survival of hospitals depends upon conforming to the DRG regulations even though some aspects of patients' safety may be compromised. Public hearings on the effects of the DRG (Bauknecht, 1985), as well as our own observations, indicate that increasing numbers of patients who are in unstable states are prematurely and improperly discharged from the hospital (Auerbach, 1985; Estes and Lee, 1986). Patients are sent home "quicker and sicker." Then, along with the cutbacks in funds to community-based health resources, in keeping with a tightening of the national budget, families are additionally burdened with the care of their ill members. Hospital nurses who must discharge these still unstable patients comment about the situation as "downright inhumane." Community-based health agencies are pressed beyond their limits (Auerbach, 1985; Taylor, 1985), with little likelihood for any increased funding. In essence, trajectory safety work has been inappropriately shifted to the family members by the DRG legislation, for they are the unpaid workers. This raises the possibility that increased rehospitalization will occur in order to rectify the mismanaged safety and/or that the rate at which illnesses stabilize will become much slower.

Hospital and community-based health agencies, now pressed to remain financially solvent, are becoming increasingly selective of their clients, giving higher preference to those who have sufficient insurance coverage or those with disease conditions of brief course. More cases are being reported where hospitals are refusing patients who have complicated, chronic illness conditions. Patients who are "medically indigent"—those not poor enough to be on welfare but not rich enough to have medicare or medicaid—are refused care in private hospitals, even in emergencies. These patients are dumped on public hospitals that are already suffering from tight budgets. Understandably, these practices have sharply raised the issue of equity of care (American Civil Liberties Union, 1986).

Despite the hardships they have created, hospital administrators and staff have attempted to live with these regulations as best they can. Health professionals have had to learn the language of business embodied in the DRGs very quickly. Assisted by such guides as *DRGs: What They Are and How to Survive Them* (Caterinicchio, 1984), they have learned to interpret the diagnostic groups and to manipulate them for more advantageous reimbursement (Simborg, 1981).

Prior to the DRGs, although sectors of health care clinicians and hospital administrators had called for better coordination of services and greater accountability in the delivery of quality care, the response by health professionals had been slow. The regulations of the DRGs have spurred intense activities, such as the development of tools to determine levels of patient's acuity of illness in order to allocate nursing resources (Schroeder, Rhodes, and Shields, 1984). Clinicians have been forced to critically examine and establish criteria on which to base standards of care for the various disease categories within the hospitalization limits. Though in general the health professionals perhaps view the DRGs negatively, some have attempted to use them positively. For instance, some nurses see the regulations as providing an opportunity for building a data base to predict the necessary nursing resources and to clarify the role of nursing in acute care hospitals (Thompson and Driers, 1985). Thus, the DRGs are seen as an opportunity to expand the role of nurses. For the most part, nurses are finding that they carry the major burden of cost-containment efforts (Selby, 1986). Traditionally, they have been the "jacks-of-all-trades." Hence, when cost cutbacks occur, they are the likely candidates for absorbing either new jobs or ones usually done by others who now have been laid off. Also, nurses working in inpatient units complain bitterly about having little time now to teach patients about their proper care before discharge, and clinics are inundated with sicker patients—but again with strained resources.

In sum, trajectory safety is subject to disruptions arising from other disruptions occurring at the administrative level, brought about by social forces outside of the hospital. In turn, a disruption at the care delivery level can contribute to disarticulation of safety policies at the administrative level, as well as to the governmental and regulatory agencies outside the hospital. There is a constant disarticulation and attempted rearticulation between the various sources of disruption. Diagrammatically the relationship is illustrated in Figure 2. The levels of safety work and the sources of disruptions are not linearly related but exist in a complex circular relationship. The safety work processes and the lines of safety work are intensively interactive. So are the factors external to the hospital, which influence matters concerning both the available resources and the legal, equity, and moral-ethical issues. The confounding aspect of this circularity is that articulation work must occur under conditions of great uncertainty.

Articulation and Rearticulation: Conditions, Strategies, and Processes

Despite all the sources of disrupted safety work, the majority of patients, of course, leave hospitals in a less hazardous physical state than when they entered. What furthers the articulating of safety work is a very powerful condition: clinical safety has major priority. This is because acute care hospitals are primarily organized around diagnosis and treatment of illnesses, some part of which is actually or potentially dangerous. Consequently, there is a concerned effort to articulate those tasks that are related to the assessing, monitoring, and rectifying of major clinical hazards. This work is articulated through accountability, whereas those tasks defined as more minor are not as carefully or explicitly articulated.

It is true that clinical safety may conflict with legal and financial considerations, with patients' comfort or identity con-

Figure 2. Interactions in Disarticulation.

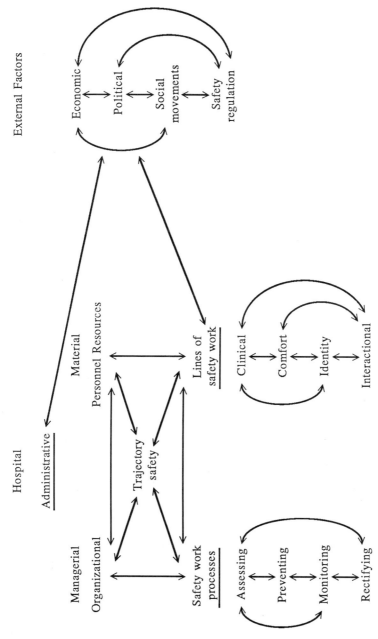

cerns, with the staff's sense of identity, or with organizational or
staff-staff relations—which may contribute to the disarticulation
of clinical safety. However, concern for clinical safety assures that
when comfort or identity tasks are important for getting a clinical
job done, then they get built into the clinical task structure.

The staff's dominant concern for clinical safety is also evident in their usual tendency to make subordinate any issues pertaining to the hospital's financial safety. This is especially true
when major clinical hazards are involved. Staff who consider
their own personal safety concerns before clinical safety, thereby
endangering patients, are severely criticized on moral grounds.
Indeed, clincial safety, along with legal safety, is a powerful
leverage in fostering articulation through explicit accountability, even in the face of hospital administrators' financial concerns. Recollect, for instance, our previous illustration that when
nurses on an ICU were unable adequately to articulate safety
work because old cardiac monitors frequently broke down and
were not replaced by the hospital administration for financial
reasons, they were able to negotiate successfully for new monitors. They did this by using the combined leverage of clinical
and legal hazards. Their arguments for new monitors listed the
clinical risks that were linked with potential legal risks, as well
as the amount of time and money lost in repairs. (They listed
lowered staff morale only as a last item.) It is unlikely that any
hospital administrator would endanger clinical and legal safety
in order to lessen financial risk. Or again, a physician who was
a member of a committee for allocating hospital resources remarked that he was troubled by the demands of the respiratory
therapy department. However, he was loath to pursue this,
both because he did not understand the technical issues involved
and because he recognized that this department dealt with lifesaving machines. He did not wish to jeopardize that department's management of major clinical hazards.

Another powerful factor in favor of articulation is that
the patients also give major priority to clinical safety. A patient
can be angry about discomforts or staff's impersonality but will
forgive the personnel because of the personnel's apparent concern with clinical safety. Interpersonal incompetence is forgivable

providing they are clinically competent, but clinical incompetence is unforgivable.

Safety articulation is constantly under review and changing, because new technologies and new kinds of trajectories require controlling the associated hazards. Thus, some aspects of
safety work are well articulated, while others lag behind in articulation. In general, articulation is related to trajectory phases
and also to phases of equipment use. In the early phases of either,
there is concerted effort to identify the major and minor hazards
that might arise; the safety limits and the criteria for assessing,
monitoring, preventing, and rectifying them; and the necessary
skill for doing these safety jobs. Where the probability of serious
hazards is high, generally there is great vigilance concerning
safety work details. Through experience, along with trial and
error, unexpected hazards are identified and evaluated. Later
they become items more precisely to be assessed, monitored,
and prevented. Consequently then, there are fewer major hazards requiring rectification, and attention can be directed to controlling the minor hazards.

Eventually, the necessary resources, the safety lines of
work, and the various safety tasks become precisely identified
and articulated in a clear task structure. Many safety tasks
become routinized, and the organizational procedures covering task sequences are developed. This enables the teaching of
these tasks. Tasks concerning safety information to be given to
patients and family are programmed. Clinical hazards usually
get first priority. When these are controlled, then matters related
to patient identity are identified and eventually become articulated into the safety task structure. In essence, when uncontrolled hazards can be anticipated, and correctly assessed and
monitored, then they are defined as preventable—providing,
of course, the necessary means are available. Thus, rationalizing of safety work and its articulation is greatest at the phase
when hazards are defined as preventable. This can be illustrated
by a potentially hazardous interaction, cardiac bypass surgery.
A decade ago patients spent two to three weeks in the hospital
with several days in the ICU. Today the usual hospital stay is
usually one week with ICU care requiring one to two days.

Informational articulation is another major type of the total work that maximizes safety. Part of this is highly routinized, like the reporting from one shift to another of safety work that has been accomplished in contrast to that requiring further attention. To avoid omissions of information, each shift member may even tape record the information, a practice becoming rapidly accepted in many large hospitals. Also, the key kinds of hazard information that must be transmitted within the team are taught. As hazards become identified and controlled, special recording forms are developed, so that relevant observations and measures can be assessed and monitored. In fact, such forms are proliferating, so that special hospital committees evaluate and standardize these forms. Of course, the legal risk of improper transmission and recording of information is an incentive for accurate record keeping and for its transmission.

Some safety tasks are common to many clinical procedures, and some hazards are common to many kinds of trajectories. Hence, there are industrial companies that produce a host of standardized informational labels to alert staff to safety tasks and to how safety disarticulation can be avoided. These labels are plastered on patients' charts and beds. They include "No breakfast," "Nothing by mouth," "Allergic to_____," "Keep head elevated," "Attention, doctor, reorder pain drug," and "Patient has pacemaker."

Specific hazards may eventually be discovered to be frequently occurring throughout the hospital. Then organization-wide arrangements are made to control them. Examples of such arrangements are infectious disease control, product evaluation, and the development of quality control mechanisms. Of course, various types of crisis teams are also formed to handle major hazards. When the control of hazards is particularly complicated, as when several departments are involved, then special intra-departmental articulators ("liaison" positions) and standing committees are created.

Aside from the special articulators, every staff person is actually a safety articulator. Of course, the range of what each articulates may be narrow or wide, and safety articulation may be an implicit or explicit part of his or her work. However, since the work processes overlap and cross several levels of workers, major and recurring disarticulations usually get picked up.

The rearticulation of disrupted safety work will, of course, vary in character with the complexity of the work and the numbers of levels (task, trajectory, organization, and managerial) that are involved in the disruption. Rearticulation generally involves much reassessing, remonitoring, and rerectifying. First, there is the identifying of what went wrong and the assessing of factors that may have contributed to the disarticulation. Discovering the disarticulation may be easy or very difficult. Having discovered the source of the disruption, solutions must be found. These must be assessed for their feasibility and appropriateness, and the appropriate work rearrangement decided upon. The balancing of risks may be an issue too, when several risks are involved. Having decided on a course of action, the new items or new work processes will be monitored, and the course of action then reassessed again. Inadequacies either in the work processes or its articulation are rectified, then remonitored and reassessed until mutual agreement (always at least an incipiently "political" process) among all involved parties is reached. This process is a continual one because any new condition may to some degree disrupt the safety work.

Let us look now at two widespread organizational strategies that have had some bearing on articulation in relation to clinical safety. Under the rubrics of "quality assurance" and "risk management," hospital management personnel and health practitioners began seriously to concern themselves with developing greater accountability in order to improve care. This concern began in the late 1970s and was greatly accelerated in the 1980s as a consquence of the DRG legislation. However, a rather curious aspect of quality assurance and risk management is their separation. *Quality care* is defined by Donabedian (1978, p. 857), a proponent of quality assurance, as "the optimal achievable result for each patient, the avoidance of physician-induced (iatrogenic) complications, and the attention to the patients and family needs in a manner that is both cost effective and reasonably documented." Clinical safety is implicitly implied in this definition. Likewise, safety is implicit in quality assurance—

that it is the implementation of a systematic evaluation mechanism to assure that the delivered care is at the optimum achievable level. The term *risk management* refers to the identification, assessment, and implementation of institutional mechanisms for managing environmental, legal, and cost risks. Proponents of risk management state that it is linked with quality care. Although risk management has been the sole concern of administrators it should be the concern of everyone (Monagle, 1980). The language used in guidelines for risk management also implicitly implies safety.

There are also the PSRO guidelines, the Joint Commission on Accreditation of Hospitals, and also the "how-to" aids. Through these, a variety of activities have been undertaken to establish greater organizational accountability for improving care. These include the establishment of standards of care and criteria for evaluating care. Other activities are related to establishing organizational structure and work processes in order to avoid confusion of work responsibilities, broken lines of communication, and other organizational flaws and deficiencies. There have been efforts to identify appropriate kinds of personnel for performing given tasks and to develop approaches for assuring the proper orientation of new workers to their job responsibilities. Efforts are also made to improve peer review mechanisms and establish mechanisms to trace and correct errors. The difficulties encountered in correcting patient care processes flow from the hospital structure itself, which separates the governing body from both administration and the medical staff, plus deficiencies in the decision-making processes. The peer review mechanisms have not been well structured and disciplined (Weinberg, 1982). Other difficulties have been an overly legalistic approach and the failure to use persuasion and to establish mechanisms of formal intervention when necessary (Thompson, 1982).

In the context of our discussion, much of the effort to achieve quality assurance is to rationalize clinical safety work. The deficiencies stem from difficulties in the integration of the various parts of the hospital structure and the alignment of safety lines of work (medical-administration). Sang-O (1984), in his review of the organizational literature on quality control, points out that while there have been thousands of studies related to standards and criteria of clinical practice and tools to evaluate clinical practice, nevertheless studies related to coordination, control, and integration have been sparse. The one relevant study was done in 1974 by Longest. This researcher's categories of coordination included those that were corrective, preventive, regulatory, and promotional. *Corrective* refers to the coordinating activities that rectify, after an error or dysfunction is discovered. *Preventive* means activities for preventing potential anticipated risks. *Regulatory* includes activities for maintaining those coordinated activities already in place. *Promotional* refers to those activities for improving coordination. This study found that coordinating activities that were promotional and preventive were most relevant to quality care. The least favorable activities were the corrective. In terms of our perspective on safety work and its articulation, the supra-articulation process includes activities related to rectifying, preventing, monitoring (regulatory), and reassessing/representing (promotional). It is our observation that carrying out coordinating activities after an error has been made is often cumbersome and is the most threatening form of safety work to staff.

The importance of greater accountability in integrating safety work processes is illustrated by another study (Knaus, Draper, Wagner, and Zimmerman, 1986), in which the performances of intensive care units in fifteen major medical centers were evaluated. The best-performing hospital had a lower death rate than predicted. The hospital with the lowest performance had a higher death rate than predicted. The key difference between them was the degree of accountability and integration of their safety work (our categorization) and the communication between health team members. The best-performing hospital had the most comprehensive nursing educational support system, with experienced master's-prepared clinical specialists whose primary responsibility was the orientation and development of nursing staff. They had the responsibility, too, for designing care protocol for the units. They also had a policy of facilitating communication between doctors and nurses on matters related to admission of patients and treatment decisions. Daily rounds of patients included house staff, attending staff, and nurses. This particular hospital was the only one that had a policy of consulting the nurse about admissions to major elective surgery, so that decisions about cancelling surgery could be made if the nursing resources were assessed as inadequate.

The least effective hospital lacked a comprehensive nursing organization and an educational program. There were no routine policies where the health team might discuss patient care problems. There were frequent disagreements about the ability of the nursing staff to treat additional patients. The staff shortages meant care was given by nurses who were not trained in ICU procedures. There was also an atmosphere of distrust between physicians and nurses.

Summary

The assurance of trajectory safety ultimately rests on a suprawork process: the complex articulation of safety work processes and lines of safety work, engaged in by many levels of workers, including administrators and care deliverers. Effective articulation rests on the degree to which the safety work can be rationalized. In this chapter, we first examined the efforts of hospitals to utilize the industrial production model in order to rationalize and articulate work. This direction of effort is fortified by the hospitals' need to remain financially solvent in the face of current cutbacks in governmental financial assistance and governmental regulations, which are themselves based on an industrial production model. The grave limitations of this model when applied to safety work was then examined. Second, we examined the difficulties encountered in rationalizing safety work because of the many disarticulating conditions derived from both the hospital's structure and sources external to the hospital. Third, the efforts of hospital workers to rationalize and articulate safety work despite the many disruptions were discussed. To do this calls for a continued process of reassessment, as disruptions occur, and then rearticulation. An overriding condition that enables articulation to occur despite the many potential and actual disparatenesses is that patients, clinicians, and administrators all recognize that safety is of primary importance. This leads to various organizational mechanisms to maximize effective articulation. Finally, quality assurance and risk management were discussed as organizational strategies that have important consequences for clinical safety.

9

⌘⌘⌘⌘⌘⌘⌘⌘⌘⌘⌘⌘⌘⌘⌘⌘⌘⌘⌘⌘⌘⌘⌘⌘

Implications for Delivering
Safe and Humane Care

Hospitals are most unusual organizations, for almost no other type of organization is organized so centrally around the issue of safety. The centrality of safety work in acute care hospitals arises from their primary rationale: to bring patients who are endangered by their illnesses to as successful as possible treatment outcomes, and in this process to inflict a minimum of harm—most particularly, to do this with a minimum of errors. Given the several types and sources of hazards associated with medical technologies, along with the ethical and legal mandates governing the practice of health care professionals for assuring quality care, safety work is virtually always in the forefront of staff attention.

In the foregoing chapters, we have examined safety issues from an organizational-work-interactional perspective. Our concept of illness trajectory links the illness course with staff work and interaction, within a complex medical technological/hospital structure context. We have in this book also touched on safety in relation to such issues as ethical and legal mandates, dehumanization, technological assessment, and equity. In short, we have attempted to show generally, and often specifically, why the ensuring of clinical safety is such a complicated, difficult enterprise.

Nevertheless, most patients leave the hospital without harm. So, one of the fundamental questions that had to be answered was: How is that possible, given the many sources of hazard and the many conditions that can go wrong in hospitals? Obviously, many things in acute care hospitals are done right. Throughout the organization, everyone understands that potential hazards are everywhere and takes care to guard against them. For the most part, too, health professionals during their training have internalized the norm of "do no harm to the patient." We have also emphasized that various organizational mechanisms and staff strategies maximize chances that "no harm" will occur. Yet when this actually happens—often through the making of errors—then the consequences can be great. Besides the clinical harm, there is the potential damage to the identity of the person who has committed the error and who possibly may lose his or her job. The reputation of the hospital may suffer since this can lead to loss of public trust. Of course, there can be financial and legal damage.

Although there are many organizational mechanisms that maximize safety, sometimes they can be ineffective because there is no unifying framework for personnel to link the managerial and the care delivery levels of the hospital. Practitioners assume that management is primarily concerned with issues of environmental safety and especially legal and cost safety, while the clinicians see their major responsibility as one of clinical safety. Hence a specific hazard prevention mechanism is not organizationally in place. As a consequence of this, safety arrangements are made defensively—after legal negligence has been found or in response to regulatory legislation.

Indeed, perhaps the central implication of our research is that there is a need for a much more integrated approach to the management of clinical safety. Achievement of further integration rests, we believe, on two essential steps. The first is an improvement of accountability in safety matters. Though it is the staff members who are actually accountable, ultimately accountability is an organizational matter. This, in turn, implies a dynamic and interactional view of hospital organization and its implicated work. So a second step in achieving flexible and integrated safety work is to understand the kinds of phenomena discussed throughout this book.

Difficulties in Maintaining Safety Accountability

Before discussing the broader clinical implications of this book, it is appropriate to discuss some of the organizational factors that act as barriers to a more unified safety organizational structure.

Safety Accountability Is Organizational Accountability. The organization of hospitals, involving as it does the numerous service departments and the many types of personnel, poses especially difficult problems for maintaining safety accountability. Each occupation, department, or service tends to view its hazard/ safety concerns as unique, and some of them are. Yet, as noted throughout this book, the complex nature of safety work both at the task and trajectory levels calls for much sharing and overlapping of safety work done among the various services and departments and by different types of personnel. Furthermore, each may be balancing hazards quite differently.

A central issue involved in safety work is related to both occupational control and occupational prerogatives. Each occupation inevitably attempts to control its own destiny—to define its own practices and to control those of its members (Freidson, 1986). Occupations train their neophytes in proper skills to carry out their work safely and to minimize the probabilities of their making mistakes. Occupations, and especially professions, tend to build rationales, collective defenses against outsiders, and the right to define standards of practice and their own mistakes (Hughes, 1971). In safety terms, these efforts are essentially directed at protecting the occupation's identity and its preferred modes of work.

In the past decades there has been an increase in articles bemoaning the continued imposition of government regulations that govern the practice of health professionals. This is said to have had detrimental effects on patient care. These critics call for more self-regulation of health workers, not only for the patient's safety but for group survival (Blair and Rubin, 1980; Peplau, 1985). Typically, the solutions offered stem from the author's own occupational perspectives. Most recommendations include improve technical training and establish more accountable criteria for safe practice concerning the various disease conditions upon which surveillance can be established. While commendable, these recommendations overlook many of the sources of error that we discussed in Chapter Five on error work. The difficulties encountered in interprofessional and intraprofessional interactions concerning errors pose great problems for both error management and group surveillance. These are largely derived from the complex interplay of illness, technology, and hospital organization. In addition, groups outside the hospital that are concerned with economic or legal issues, equity, or standards of care, will continue to press their views about what is judged to be professional prerogative. As we have frequently noted, these concerns are directly or indirectly linked with some aspect of patient safety.

The establishing of organizational accountability for safety, then, necessitates interactions and negotiations that are not only interprofessional but involve groups outside of the hospital. Yet there is a relative incapacity of trained health professionals to solve problems that are essentially organizational problems by thinking in genuinely organizational terms. (That is perhaps why there is so much complaint about the "lack of communication" and the need for interprofessional communication.) Health practitioners' training is overwhelmingly focused on clinical-technical matters. They are not trained to analyze social processes, such as role making and negotiation, or the nature and operations of complex organizations (Becker, Geer, Hughes, and Strauss, 1961; Olesen and Whittaker, 1968; Coombs, 1978; Bosk, 1979; Light, 1980). Although practitioners certainly come to develop insights in these areas based on personal experience, they do not formalize their knowledge or systematically share it. Practitioners are concerned with solving technical problems and do not especially focus on social structure or the interprofessional processes through which their clinical business is conducted (Garfinkel, 1967). This situation is especially true among physicians, but to a lesser degree among nurses.

Discrepancies Between Administrators' and Clinicians' Perspectives. There is another set of conditions that perhaps hinders effective organizational accountability: the goals of hospital administrators are sometimes in competition with the goals of health practitioners. As noted in the previous chapter, hospitals are moving increasingly toward an industrial production model in order to contain costs. This movement has been hastened as a consequence of the DRG legislation. As an instance of discrepancies between administrative and clinical perspectives, we shall examine the language and assumptions of the DRG legislation.

We fully recognize that there must be efficient fiscal accounting and monitoring systems for containing the costs of acute care and that many economic abuses have been made by hospitals and care givers, thus contributing to spiraling costs. It is also true that prospective reimbursement approaches have some merit for assuring fiscal and clinical accountability. Nevertheless, the limitations of the DRG approach become more apparent when seen from the standpoint of chronic illness.

Interest groups that are undoubtedly most involved with or support the DRG regulations include the most cost-conscious: government officials, economists, hospital administrators, and corporation executives whose employees' health benefits continue to rise yearly and who feel grossly hampered by care providers' resistance to containment of costs. The very language of the DRG regulations reflects the industrial model, which we would expect these groups to favor. The DRG advocates naturally think in terms of a "health industry," one composed of many firms (hospitals) producing varied products (medical care). This industrial model is designed to rationalize work to assure minimal financial loss through well-defined goals and efficient accounting and monitoring systems and rational work processes. Quotations from the key article by the sources (Fetter and others, 1980) for this legislation make this perspective very apparent.

> The major function of an acute-care inpatient facility is to provide the diagnostic and therapeutic service required by physicians in the clinical management of their patient. Considered as an entity, the hospital's outputs are the specific services it provides in terms of hours of nursing care, medications and laboratory tests. Its inputs are the labor,

material and equipment used in the provision of
these services which is referred to here as a product of the hospital—since individual patients receive different amounts and types of services, the
hospital may be viewed as a multi-product firm with
a product line that in theory is as extensive as the
number of patients it services. The particular product provided each patient is dependent upon his
condition as well as the treatment process he under-
goes during his stay.

The fundamental purpose of the DRG approach is to identify in the acute care setting a set
of case types, each representing a class of patients
with similar processes of care and predictable packages of services (or product) from an institution. . . .
in order to evaluate, compare, and provide relevant feedback regarding hospital performance, it
is necessary to identify the specific product that institutions provide (p. 12).

This industrial imagery is explicitly focused on patients'
diseases rather than on patients themselves. Patients are seen
as consumers—they pay for produced products; they are sur-
rogates for them. Clinicians have difficulty with this imagery
since they always see diseases in terms of patients (this despite
those clinicians who refer impersonally to "the cardiac patient
in Room 101"). They also recognize that patients often impede
the rational application of medical techniques.

An underlying assumption made by the DRG proponents
is that there are predictable packages of services (medical interventions based on rational work processes) and that their
"outputs" are predictable. Although it is true that many illnesses
are characterized by a predictable package of services and outcomes, the dominance of today's prevalent chronic illnesses
makes a totally rational, predictable service very difficult to
achieve. As indicated in our discussion of risk assessment and
trajectory safety, many medical interventions and their consequences are highly uncertain and unclear. Given the wide varie-

ties of treatment options, there are lively debates among clinicians as to the respective risk benefits and also the appropriateness of different interventions for different illness phases. Given the complexity of treatment task structures and the possibility of unexpected contingencies disrupting the treatment work processes, the rationalization of important aspects of treatment work is rendered quite problematic (Strauss, Fagerhaugh, Suczek, and Wiener, 1985).

The medical-industrial model attempts to rationalize medical services by focusing only on the diseases and their severity, but the reality is that consumers demand humane and safe medical services for managing diseases. But alas, humane service is hard to quantify. Outcomes of medical service ultimately rest on hazard/safety work done throughout the production process, and there is not, and cannot be, complete agreement about the efficiency or risk/benefits of many of the treatment options. Outcomes are almost always determined in terms of weighing and balancing benefits and risks, but quantification of this is extremely difficult. Hence, the rationalizing of medical services can only apply to those diseases that have a short course and can be managed during the hospitalization itself.

Let us be purposely ironic and paraphrase, as a hypothetical business administrator might, the central clinical safety concerns of hospital staffs: "The overall goal of acute care hospitals is to diagnose, palliate, and treat consumers endangered by diseases. However, both the medical products (diagnostic and treatment procedures) and the providers of care in the production process are potential—sometimes probable—sources of hazards for the endangered consumers. The production process (division of labor and organization of work tasks) must always take safety work (assessing, monitoring, preventing, and rectifying potential hazards) into account. Outcomes are based on (1) how efficiently and effectively the consumers have been managed throughout the work processes, with a minimum of physical and psychological harm and 2) the degree to which the consumers are finally out of danger. (And, we might add, free of the potential risks of medical interventions.)"

However, in terms of our own terminology, the staff's giving of quality care sums up to establishing and coordinating lines of work and lines of communication among multiple workers, both laterally and hierarchically. Thus, problems related to safety can be resolved in the service of quality assurance. Also included is the cooperative establishment of safety criteria through which the evaluating and monitoring of work processes, organizational arrangements, and patient outcomes can be done. This establishment of criteria occurs within a context of available resources (money, materials, and personnel) and through careful consideration of the consequences of various contingencies (legal, regulations, and so on) as they might affect patients', workers', and institutional safety. Quality and safety assurance together surely make sense to clinicians, since this combination is congruent with the main goal of their work.

What safety accountability then amounts to is the building into an organization of various work arrangements and communication linkages designed to make safety more visible, precise, and associated with a responsible division of labor. Both the increasing medical specialization and the separation of clinical and support services (such as repair and maintenance of machinery) precipitate difficulties; yet the very complexity of hospitals necessitates a greater organizational accountability. Given the uncertainty inherent in many illness trajectories and the medical interventions that produce new ones, the safety arrangements must be flexible in order to respond successfully to the constantly changing contingencies and the new safety concerns.

In short, once these matters are understood analytically—that is, in conceptual terms and not just experientially—then staffs can build the more integrated approach to safety that is so obviously needed today.

Clinical Implications and Policy Suggestions

Our perspective points to a multifaceted approach that takes into account not only the patient's physical and psychosocial safety but also the safety of workers and the hospital. No

doubt there are various clinical implications that readers themselves will draw from the detailed discussions of previous chapters. Based on our approach and its many implications, we shall
conclude now with several organizationally oriented suggestions.

Need for Stable, Trained Staff. To begin with, the hospital
personnel can be sources of hazard. Therefore, efforts should
be continued to assure that they are performing safely and
reliably. Orientation programs for new workers and educational
programs to upgrade skills should be strengthened to meet the
constantly changing safety needs. Practical efforts, such as men-
tor programs where experienced practitioners assist newcomers
to gain the necessary skill and knowledge, should be encouraged.

Much effective organizational accountability comes about
as a result of personnel working together for long periods of time.
Their collective experiential knowledge about safety issues eventually evolves into accepted norms of work. An essential part
of organizational accountability, therefore, consists of encouraging workers' stability. This tends to maximize open discussion
even across occupational lines, in the service of improving safe,
humane care. Since experiential knowledge is of primary importance, it is useful to identify how experts develop the art of
expertise. Studies to identify this seem a fruitful way to learn
how to develop expertise in others and how to teach these skills
to novices (Benner, 1984; Benner and Tanner, 1987). However,
a stable work force depends upon discovering ways to assess,
monitor, and rectify the potential burnout of staff before it is
too late—and personnel do quit their jobs (Buechler, 1985; Cherniss, 1980; McConnell, 1982).

Need for Negotiation and Shared Power. In the communication that is so necessary today, skills at negotiation are essential for resolving differences and for reaching consensus. This
requires learning ways of improving interdisciplinary communication. Yet this is not easy to achieve because of a lack of role
clarity and incongruent expectations, as well as differences in
authority, power, status, autonomy, educational preparation,
and personality characteristics (Given and Simon, 1977; Nagi,
1975). Open discussion requires at least partially overcoming
these barriers. Nurses in particular feel these keenly because
not only are they on the front lines of care but their work depends

very much upon the coordination of work done by many other workers. Hence nurses have attempted to cope with these barriers by discussion and by learning how to gain some measure of influence without antagonizing others, especially those of higher status. The training of middle-management nurses emphasizes how to resolve conflicts and issues involved in decision making, how to affect change, and how to function within an interdisciplinary team (Booth, 1983; Brill, 1976; Chater, 1983; Del Bruno, 1986; Ducanis and Golis, 1979). If only in terms of maximizing clincial safety, there is a need to equalize power within the health team. Physicians who practice in hospitals must, we suggest, learn how to share power in the service both of their own treatment goals and in the interests of their patients' maximal safety.

It is interesting to note that the quality circle approach used in Japanese industry is now being proposed as a possible solution for problems in American health care organizations (Cornell, 1984; Fitzgerald and Murphy, 1982; Orlikoff and Snow, 1984). Proponents of the quality circle approach argue that our own system of work organization emphasizes individualism, status lines, competitiveness, economic growth, and short-term profit but minimizes discussion in decision making (Adair, Fitzgerald, Nygard, and Shaffer, 1982; Fitzgerald and Murphy, 1982). In contrast, the quality circle approach emphasizes collective and collaborative action, building competence, and maximizing discussion for decision making, while deemphasizing status. However, some critics urge caution, noting that hospitals may be, as in the past, looking for a new miracle drug and so will be disappointed; middle-management administrators have gone through too many fads, such as flex time and management by objectives (McKinney, 1984). Suffice it to say that this interest in quality circles flows from an understandable desire to find genuinely accountable ways to resolve the hospital's many complex problems.

Need for Open Discussion of Errors. Error management is also crucial to safety accountability. Indeed, it is through the occurrence of errors that shortcomings in skills, resources, and work processes are likely to become visible. As discussed in Chapter Five, all too often errors are discussed among clinicians only in terms of legal or financial risk and error, or in terms of blame. Because interactions around safety issues are very delicate and threatening there is little open discussion about errors, especially of those related to regulations and the surveillance of incompetent colleagues. Perusal of books about hospital administration shows little discussion of error management. Quite often the topic is buried within chapters related to "human relations and administration." For staff to be able to handle errors accountably, however, requires opportunities for them to discuss errors openly and critically, to gain group support, and to find ways of improving both their error management and their interactions with respect to errors. Open discussion is also necessary with the public, but communication with the public is made more difficult if open discussion is not occurring within the professional groups. Furthermore, the complexity of care and the uncertainty attending the use of medical technologies mean that infallibility and the errorless imperative are almost impossible to attain. This makes openness with the public about errors still more urgent. As long as error is thought of in terms of blame, the staff's interaction can readily deteriorate into defensive maneuvering, involving coercion or other types of unproductive interaction. Blaming prevents discussion, negotiation, persuasion, and teaching—the more positive ways of resolving this very complex problem, which is so central to maximizing clinical safety.

Concept of Trajectory Safety Versus Acute Care Model

Emphasized throughout these pages have been the linkages among several medical technology-related issues (risk/benefit, cost, moral/ethical, equity, dehumanization), as well as how these issues are hotly debated both inside and outside the hospital. Health policies that fail to take this into account can have far-reaching negative consequences for clinical safety, given the prevalence of patients with chronic illness in hospitals today.

Although we have focused primarily on hazard/safety as related to acute and highly unstable phases of illness, our concept of trajectory safety implies more than just acute phases and a clinical emphasis. The concept takes into account the complex interactions of clinical, comfort, and identity safety throughout the various phases of the illness. After all, trajectory safety issues extend over the course of an illness. Persons with chronic illnesses have varying patterns of acute and stable phases (also unstable, comeback, deteriorating, and dying phases). Over the course of an illness, the site of safety management can shift from acute care hospital to home (often in cycles) or to other care facilities (rehabilitation, long-term care, hospices, and so on). While at home, the ill and kin are largely responsible for clinical safety. How effectively they carry out that work depends upon how effectively hospital workers provide them with the necessary information and skills to do this work and how effectively, in turn, they link these with appropriate resources outside the hospital (home and health care services). When the number of resources and/or their articulation is insufficient, then the likelihood of an acute phase increases. When health care policies emphasize one phase without much regard to other phases, then overall trajectory safety is jeopardized.

American health policies have focused primarily on the acute (hospital) phase, without an awareness of how this policy affects other phases experienced by the ill over the long haul (Corbin and Strauss, forthcoming a). This parochial perspective results in chaotic health care delivery, as well as tensions and anger among health care providers inside and outside the hospital (Lubkin, 1986). In addition, it increases angry confrontation by advocacy groups that is linked with medical technology-related issues. The advocates usually see only one of the linked issues—the one they themselves value (Wiener, Fagerhaugh, Strauss, and Suczek, 1982). This means that the cost focus taken almost wholly by itself in relation to acute care hospitals is senseless; costs must be considered in terms of a long view of trajectory safety. We must take seriously that it is chronic illnesses that are being treated.

Need for Public Awareness and Open Discussion

Both the public and the health practitioners desire safe, humane health services. The public needs to be better informed about the complexity of health care, including the issue of safety, and the broader social and economic issues intertwined with care. There is a strong tendency toward adversarial relationships by consumer advocates and among industrial and professional groups; however, mutual understanding and respect for one another's problems is becoming increasingly crucial—certainly with regard to safety issues. Yet unless the self-serving strategies of various participants are mitigated, the health care system will doubtless continue in its present state of conflict.

Over the last decade the credibility of health professionals seems to have declined somewhat among the public. That medicine is not infallible, or treatments always safe, is being recognized. More and more people are no longer willing to accept the belief that only the health professionals are capable of understanding the complex and technical issues of health care. So there is now increasing public discussion and debate on these issues.

Yet it would be well if the public, as well as the health professionals, would understand that safety, medical technology, costs/benefits, legal matters, morality, and dehumanization are tightly linked issues, along with the complex weighing and balancing of risk benefits in finding solutions to the many health care problems, and the issue of who benefits and who bears the risks of given actions. We all need to know more about the risk consequences of health policy changes and the risks entailed in adopting new technologies. Jennett, a British neurologist (1986) familiar with both British and American health systems, urges American physicians to engage more vigorously in technological assessments but points out that cost/benefit and equity are related issues. He, too, urges more open public discussion.

Health professionals could also utilize the media with greater responsibility. In recent years an increasing number of media programs have given information about how to take care of bodies so as to prevent disease and how to manage chronic illnesses; of course, this focus is commendable. However, there is relatively little discussion of the pressing issues that have been addressed in this book—including the risks associated with interventions—issues that cannot be resolved without an informed public.

Too often media reporting consists of creating public relations events. Perhaps the most blatant were the series of events concerning the Jarvik artificial heart, when the public was bombarded daily about the patient's progress or lack of progress. Because the artificial heart was (and still is) highly experimental, controversial, and costly, health professionals were privately discussing among themselves the safety, risk/benefit, moral, and cost/benefit issues. Yet this discussion was not made public. Government officials and even the president of the United States used this surgical operation for public relations purposes (making congratulatory telephone calls and so on). Meanwhile, these same officials were drastically cutting funds for many crucial medical and illness preventive services.

In closing, it is appropriate to return again to think about safety specifically as safety along the entire course of a trajectory—that is what makes the difference. Acute care hospitals are focused primarily on lifesaving and decreasing the danger to a manageable level. At home, however, patients and their families carry the major burden of keeping the trajectories stable and attempting to prevent medical crises by adhering to various medical regimens. In doing so, they do all the necessary safety work. And the amount of this work is truly enormous, for the safety work that is pertinent to illness management at home is all intertwined with the work of living (Corbin and Strauss, 1985, and forthcoming b). Contingencies that affect living (like having a child with the flu, getting sick, losing a job, or even having the hot water heater go out) can upset the clinical safety work. Trajectories that are going downhill, with alternating phases of increasing deterioration and then stability, impede or make the safety work difficult. Of course, contingencies that disrupt trajectory safety in hospitals are frequent, but there are incomparably more of these at home.

So for the further and long-range effectiveness of their own intensive efforts to ensure clinical safety, it is vital that hospital staffs thoroughly comprehend that these relate to other safety work performed continuously at home. The total safety depends upon the articulation of many lines of safety work engaged in not only by health professionals inside and outside of hospitals but on that done by the ill and their families. The ill and kin are quite aware of those relationships and how difficult is their coordination. It is the health professionals and health policymakers who need more fully to comprehend this same set of relationships and the kinds of problems faced by patients and families in carrying out safety work while living at home. This is the ultimate meaning of chronic illness for safety issues.

Summary

Perhaps the central implication of our research is that there is a need for a much more integrated approach to the management of clinical safety. The achievement of further integration rests on two essential steps: (1) an improvement of accountability for safety activities, inevitably an organizational matter and (2) understanding the kinds of phenomena discussed in the foregoing chapters. Several barriers to a more unified safety organizational structure were discussed. Among these were the strains emanating from attempts by occupations to control their work and protect their identities, with consequent breakdowns in or failures to negotiate and interact effectively in terms of ensuring clinical safety. We also discussed discrepancies between the perspectives of administrators and clinicians that affect the management of clinical safety. We pointed out what the DRG regulations and the industrial model of health care imply in this regard. We cautioned that efforts to improve safety accountability would have to deal with some of those kinds of barriers— and argued the need for building into the organization of work various arrangements and communication linkages designed to make safety more visible, precise, and associated with responsible division of labor.

We next turned to several clinical implications: the need for stable, trained staff; the need for negotiation and shared power among hospital personnel; and the need for open discussion of errors, including with the general public. We closed with policy suggestions, centering discussion around the usefulness of our concept of trajectory, in order to focus the attention of practitioners and policymakers on chronic illness as a lifetime course of illness that has various phases and combinations of phases. These take the ill in and out of various health facilities, but the work of managing illness takes place not only there but at home. Ultimately, the ensuring of clinical safety in hospitals links with and is interdependent with the safety work done at home.

Appendix

Methodological Note

The research project that produced this book and a preceding one, *The Social Organization of Medical Work* (Strauss, Fagerhaugh, Suczek, and Wiener, 1985), began in the late 1970s. That project was designed to trace the impact of medical technology, especially machines, on the work of hospital personnel when giving care to patients. The research team consisted of the four authors, who worked closely on all phases of the study. Its research style and associated modes of "grounded theory" analysis have been descibed extensively in previous publications written or co-authored by Anselm Strauss (Glaser and Strauss, 1965, 1967, 1968, 1970; Fagerhaugh and Strauss, 1977; Schatzman and Strauss, 1973; Strauss, 1970, 1986; also see Glaser, 1978). Our exploratory interviews and field observations for this project were originally carried out in 1976. The project received United States Public Health Service funding through the years from 1977 to 1981. The research design called generally for field observation on a variety of hospital wards selected at first by selective sampling (Schatzman and Strauss, 1973) and later by theoretical sampling (Glaser and Strauss, 1967; Glaser, 1978; Strauss, 1986), and also on various kinds of wards in several different kinds of hospital in order to maximize certain structural conditions: a city-county hospital, a large urban community hospital, a military hospital, a university hospital, two small urban hospitals, and a suburban community hospital.

The fieldwork was intensive and carried out by three members of the research team. In addition, a great number of open-ended interviews were conducted with hospital personnel selected in accordance with concepts and hypotheses that emerged

227

over the course of the study. Substantially fewer interviews were done with persons who represented special interests arising from our evolving research: hospital architects, hospital administrators, medical equipment innovators, designers, medical researchers, and so on. The resulting data were analyzed along the lines discussed in the above-mentioned publications. The research ultimately led in some directions not foreseen when writing the original research proposal. Thus, we began with the idea that there would be at least one book and several articles, presumably about the impact of medical equipment on patient care and perhaps on the health occupations.

We did not anticipate originally that the issue of clinical safety would be so central either to medical/nursing care or, correspondingly, to our research. Early in the project, however, we began to sense some of its importance, and so we began to code our data in terms of clinical safety and to direct some observations and interview queries to safety issues, doing this in terms of theoretical sampling and pertinent hypotheses and research questions. Eventually, we pulled together and summarized our accumulated codes and theoretical memos, discussing this summary at a long team meeting. This discussion in turn raised a number of further theoretical issues and associated lines of inquiry.

Toward the end of the project, we wrote one long paper titled "Chronic Illness, Medical Technology, and Clinical Safety in the Hospital" (Fagerhaugh, Strauss, Suczek, and Wiener, 1986). We also included a chapter on that topic in the first book published from our project. For various reasons, but principally because funding ran out and project members dispersed to do other work, the book took longer to finish than it might otherwise. In addition, we found that many important theoretical issues and conceptual details had not been worked out, because only relatively late in the project did we decide to write a separate volume about clinical safety.

One of us, Shizuko Fagerhaugh, carried the principal burden of thinking through, working out, and writing the book, but, of course, it is very much the product of the entire team's collaborative research. It is also the product of still earlier work by us in hospitals and homes, on terminal care, pain management, and chronic illness—including the use of much data, central concepts, and theoretical conceptions derived from that lengthy research program.

Perhaps a few additional words might be useful for those readers who are especially interested in methods of qualitative analysis. As noted, we used the usual grounded theory techniques—including coding and theoretical sampling—made systematic comparisons, wrote theoretical memos, and, of course, weaved back and forth between data and their interpretation. As described in the preceding book (Strauss, Fagerhaugh, Suczek, and Wiener, 1985) from this project, our weekly team meetings became essentially generating sessions for coding and theory while the transcripts of these discussions became a type of theoretical memo. When we actually got around to developing the fuller theoretical exposition laid out in this book, however, we had perforce to continue coding and memo writing. For the most part, it was not necessary to gather additional data, but it was entirely necessary to return to our accumulated data for verification of newly evolved theoretical points. The ruminations stimulated by thinking about or scrutinizing the data forced some further theoretical development. We found that we had blurred or "black-boxed" relationships needing clarification and that we needed to spell out conceptual relationships now becoming visible to us but not yet sufficiently elaborated or detailed.

Even when the first draft was essentially finished, the senior author found himself asking, but what have we left out of this picture, given what we know about the contemporary hospital's functioning, and which earlier we discussed in terms other than safety? In consequence, additional sections were added to the manuscript, such as those on information work. We also developed a much more detailed discussion of articulation work in relation to safety. If ever a publication written in the grounded theory style has departed from the suggested practice of more or less being written from accumulated theoretical memos—because all the major conceptualizations is done before embarking on the manuscript writing—this book did. In doing so, of course, it only made more evident the usual experience of, in fact, never being finished with a research report until the last lines of the last draft are written! The qualitative analysis style of research does force major conceptualizations long before the writing, and the accumulation of memos does speed up and appreciably help conceptual integration. This was all true of our research on clinical safety. Yet the special character of this aspect of our total project did also alter the usual rules of thumb. All such rules are meant, anyhow, to be helpful guides—not strict rules.

Even after a draft was submitted to the publisher, the reviewers raised several issues, which in order to answer or give more elaborate answers necessitated our going back to the library to find additional documentation (data). This search for additional data is, too, a special type of sampling of the data out there that is an integral part of data collection procedures. It is one that is rarely mentioned in methodological discussions, although presumably it is not such a rare occurrence in qualitative research.

References

Abrams, N. A. "A Contrary View of Nurse as Patient Advocate." *Nursing Forum,* 1978, *17* (1), 260–266.

Abramson, N. S., Wald, K. S., Grenvik, A.N.A., and Snyder, J. V. "Adverse Occurrences in Intensive Care Units." *Journal of American Medical Association,* 1980, *244* (14), 1582–1584.

Adair, M., Fitzgerald, M., Nygard, K., and Shaffer, F. *Quality Circle in Nursing Services.* New York: National League for Nursing, 1982.

Agarwal, S. K. "Infusion Pump Artifacts: The Potential Danger of a Spurious Dysrhythmia." *Heart and Lung,* 1980, *9* (6), 1063–1065.

Alfidid, R. J. "Controversy, Alternatives and Decisions in Complying with the Legal Doctrine of Informed Consent." *Radiology,* 1975, *14,* 231–234.

Altman, S. H., and Blandon, P. (eds.). *Medical Technology: The Culprit Behind the Health Care Cost?* Proceedings of 1977 Sun Valley Forum of National Health. Department of Health, Education and Welfare publication no. (PHS) 79-3216. Washington, D.C.: U.S. Government Printing Office, 1979.

American Civil Liberties Union, San Francisco Chapter. "Emergency Rooms Door Closing: ACLU Takes on Patient Dumping." *ACLU News,* 1986, *52,* 1–3.

American Nurses Association. *Code for Nurses with Interpretive Statements.* Kansas City, Mo.: American Nurses Association, 1979.

Andreopoulos, S. (ed.). *Primary Care: Where Medicine Fails.* New York: Wiley, 1974.

Annas, G. J., Glantz, L. H., and Katz, B. F. *Informed Consent to Human Experimentation: The Subject's Dilemma.* Cambridge, Mass.: Ballinger, 1977.

Ashley, J. A. *Hospitals, Paternalism and the Role of Nurses.* New York: Teachers College Press, 1976.

Auerbach, M. "Changes in Home Health Care Delivery." *Nursing Outlook,* 1985, *33* (6), 290–291.

Ayers, R. "Effects and Role Development in the Clinical Nurse Specialist." *Nursing Digest,* 1979, *6,* 15–21.

Bauknecht, V. L. "Testimony Cites Impact of DRG System." *American Nurse,* 1985, *17* (3), 8.

Becker, H., Geer, B., Hughes, E. C., and Strauss, A. L. *Boys in White: Student Culture in Medical School.* Chicago: University of Chicago Press, 1961.

Benner, P. *From Novice to Expert: Excellence and Power in Clinical Nursing Practice.* Reading, Mass.: Addison-Wesley, 1984.

Benner, P., and Tanner, C. "How Expert Nurses Use Intuition." *American Journal of Nursing,* 1987, *87,* 23–31.

Bennett, J. G. (ed.). "Symposium on Self-Care Concept of Nursing." *Nursing Clinics of North America,* 1980, *15* (1), 129–217.

Bierig, J. R. "Whatever Happened to Professional Self-Regulation?" *Bar Leader,* 1980, *8,* 18–20.

Blackburn, S. "Job Dissatisfaction Causes RN Shortage." *American Journal of Nursing,* 1980, *8* (9), 1527–1528.

Blackburn, S. "The Neonatal ICU: A High Risk Environment." *American Journal of Nursing,* 1982, *82* (12), 1708–1712.

Blair, P. D., and Rubin, S. (eds.). *Regulating the Professions.* Lexington, Mass.: Heath, 1980.

Booth, R. Z. "Power: A Negative and Positive Form in Relationship." *Nursing Administration Quarterly,* 1983, *7,* 10–20.

Bosk, C. L. *Forgive and Remember: Managing Medical Failure.* Chicago: University of Chicago Press, 1979.

Brill, N. J. *Teamwork: Working in the Health Services.* Philadelphia: Lippincott, 1976.

Broadhead, R. S., and Facchinetti, N. J. "Drug Iatrogenesis and Clinical Pharmacy: The Mutual Fate of Social Problems and a Professional Movement." *Social Problems,* 1985, *32,* 425–436.

Brodt, D. E. "Nursing Process." In N. Chaska (ed.), *Nursing Profession.* New York: McGraw-Hill, 1978.

Brook, R. H., William, K. N., and Avery, A. D. "Quality Assurance Today and Tomorrow: Forecast for the Future." *Annals of International Medicine,* 1976, *95,* 809–817.

Brown, B., Jr. *Risk Management for Hospitals.* Rockville, Md.: Aspen Corp., 1979.

Bucher, R., and Strauss, A. "Professions in Process." *American Journal of Sociology,* 1961, *66* (4), 325–334.

Buechler, D. K. "Help for the Burned Out Nurse." *Nursing Outlook,* 1985, *33* (4), 181–192.

Bunker, J. P., Fowles, J., and Schaffarzich, R. "Evaluation of Medical Technology Assessment." *New England Journal of Medicine,* 1981, *306,* 620–624.

Byars, D. P., and others. "Randomized Clinical Trials: Perspectives on Some Recent Ideas." *New England Journal of Medicine,* 1978, *295,* 74–80.

Byers, V. B. *Nursing Observations.* Dubuque, Iowa: Brown, 1975.

Caterinicchio, R. P. (ed.). *DRGs: What They Are and How to Survive Them.* Stack, N.J.: Thorofare, 1984.

Chang, B. L. "Evaluation of Health Care Professionals in Facilitating Self Care: Review of Literature and a Conceptual Model." *Advances in Nursing Science,* 1980, *25,* 45–88.

Chapman, J. E., and Chapman, H. H. *Behavior and Health Care: A Humanistic Helping Process.* St. Louis, Mo.: Mosby, 1975.

Charmaz, K. *The Social Reality of Death: Death in Contemporary America.* Reading, Mass.: Addison-Wesley, 1980.

Chater, S. S. "Creative Use of Power." In M. E. Connery and O. Andruski (eds.), East Norwalk, Conn.: Appleton-Century-Crofts, 1983.

Chavigny, K. H., and Helm, A. "Ethical Dilemmas and the Practice of Infection Control." *Law, Medicine and Health,* 1982, *174,* 168–170.

Cherniss, C. *Professional Burnout in Human Service Organizations.* New York: Praeger, 1980.

Christman, L. "Expansion of Nursing Practice, Moral Dilemmas for Practitioners in a Changing Society." *Nursing Digest,* 1978, *6,* 47–49.

Cleland, V. "Sex Discrimination: Nursing's Most Pervasive Problem." *American Journal of Nursing,* 1981, *81,* 1542–1547.

Coates, V. T. "Technology and Public Policy: Summary Report." Prepared for National Science Foundation. Washington, D.C.: George Washington University, 1972.

Committee for Evaluating Medical Technology in Clinical Practice, Division of Health Policy, Institute of Medicine (U.S.). *Assessing Medical Technology.* Washington, D.C.: National Academy Press, 1985.

Conway-Rutowsky, B. "Patient Participation in the Nursing Process." *The Nursing Clinics of North America,* 1982, *17,* 451–457.

Coombs, R. H. *Mastering Medicine.* New York: Free Press, 1978.

Cooper, J. B., and Covialon, L. A., Jr. *Accidental Breathing System Disconnection: Interim Report to Food and Drug Administration.* (Contract no. 233-82-5070.) Cambridge, Mass.: A. D. Little, 1983.

Corbin, J., and Strauss, A. "Managing Chronic Illness at Home: Three Lines of Work." *Qualitative Sociology,* 1985, *8* (3), 224–247.

Corbin, J., and Strauss, A. *Unheard Voices: Chronic Illness and American Health Policy.* Forthcoming a.

Corbin, J., and Strauss, A. *Unending Work and Care.* Forthcoming b.

Cornell, L. "Quality Circle a New Cure for Hospital Dysfunctions?" *Hospital and Health Service Administration,* 1984, *29,* 87–93.

Corwin, R. G. "The Professional Employee: A Study of Conflicts in Nursing Roles." *American Journal of Sociology,* 1961, *66,* 604–612.

Couch, N. P., Tilney, N. L., Rayner, A. A., and Moore, H. D. "The High Cost of Low-Frequency Events: The Anatomy of Surgical Mishaps." *New England Journal of Medicine,* 1981, *304,* 634–637.

Crozier, M. *The Bureaucratic Phenomena.* Chicago: University of Chicago Press, 1967.

Curtin, L. L., and Flaherty, M. S. *Nursing Ethics: Theories and Pragmatics.* Englewood Cliffs, N.J.: Prentice-Hall, 1982.

Cushing, M. "Legal Side: Failure to Communicate." *American Journal of Nursing*, 1982, *82* (10), 1597.

Davis, A. J., and Aroskar, M. A. *Ethical Dilemmas in Nursing Practice*. Englewood Cliffs, N.J.: Prentice-Hall, 1983.

Del Bruno, D. J. "Power and Politics in Organization." *Nursing Outlook*, 1986, *34*, 124–128.

Donabedian, A. "The Quality of Care." *Science*, 1978, *200*, 856–861.

Donahue, M. P. "The Nurse—A Patient Advocate." *Nursing Forum*, 1982, *17* (2), 149–151.

Donnelly, G. F. "The Assertive Nurse or How to Say What You Mean Without Shaking or Shouting." *Nursing*, 1978, *8*, 66–69.

Drucker, P. F. *Technology Management and Society*. New York: Harper & Row, 1970.

Ducanis, A., and Golis, A. *The Interdisciplinary Health Care Team: A Handbook*. Rockville, Md.: Aspen Corp., 1979.

Duran, G. S. "On the Scene: Risk Management in Health Care." *Nursing Administration Quarterly*, 1980, *5* (1), 19–22.

Ederer, F. "Practical Problems in Collaborative Clinical Trials." *American Journal Epidemiology*, 1975, *120*, 111–118.

Ehrenreich, B., and Ehrenreich, J. *The American Health Empire: A Report from Health Policy Advisory Center*. New York: Vantage Press, 1971.

Emerson, R., and Pollner, M. "Dirty Work Designations: Their Features and Consequence in Psychiatric Settings." *Social Problems*, 1976, *23*, 243–254.

Engel, G. L. "The Biopsychosocial Model of Education in Health Professions." *Annals of the New York Academy of Science*, 1978, *310*, 169–181.

Estes, C. L. *Long-Term Care and Public Policy in an Era of Austerity*. San Francisco: Institute of Health and Aging, 1986.

Estes, C. L., and Lee, P. R. "Health Problems and Policy Issues of Old Age." In L. Aiken and D. Mechanic (eds.), *Applications of Social Science to Clinical Medicine and Health Policy*. New Brunswick, N.J.: Rutgers University Press, 1986.

Fagerhaugh, S., and Strauss, A. *Politics of Pain Management: Patient-Staff Interaction*. Reading, Mass.: Addison-Wesley, 1977.

Fagerhaugh, S., Strauss, A., Suczek, B. and Wiener, C.
"Chronic Illness, Medical Technology, and Clinical Safety
in the Hospital." In J. Roth (ed.), *Research in the Sociology of
Health Care.* Vol. 4. Greenwich, Conn.: JAI Press, 1986.

Fagin, C. M. "Nurses' Rights." *American Journal of Nursing,*
1975, *75* (1), 52–62.

Fein, R. *Medical Care, Medical Costs: A Search for Health Insurance
Policy.* Cambridge, Mass.: Harvard University Press, 1986.

Feliu, A. G. "The Risk of Blowing the Whistle." *American Journal
of Nursing,* 1983, *83* (10), 1387–1388, 1390.

Fetter, R., and others. "Case Mix Definition by Diagnosis-
Related Groups." *Medical Care,* 1980, *18,* 1–53.

Fineberg, H. V. "Technology Assessment: Motivations, Capabilities and Future Directions." *Medical Care,* 1985, *23,* 663–
671.

Fitzgerald, L., and Murphy, J. *Installing Quality Circle: A Strategic
Approach.* San Diego, Calif.: University Associate Press, 1982.

Flaherty, M. J. "The Nurse as Advocate." *Nursing Management,*
1981, *12* (9), 12–13.

Freidson, E. *Doctoring Together: A Study of Professional Social Control.* New York: Elsevier, 1976.

Freidson, E. *Professional Competence.* Chicago: University of Chicago Press, 1986.

Freishtat, H. W. "Technology Versus Regulation." In B. J.
McNeil and E. G. Cravalho (ed.), *Critical Issues in Medical
Technology.* Boston, Mass.: Auburn House, 1982.

Frekin, V. *Technologized Man: The Myth and Reality.* New York:
George Brazillar, 1969.

Freudenberger, H. J. "Staff Burnout." *Journal of Social Issues,*
1974, *30,* 159–165.

Fuchs, V. R. "The Growing Demand for Medical Care." *New
England Journal of Medicine,* 1968, *279* (4), 190–195.

Garfinkel, H. *Studies in Ethnomethodology.* Englewood Cliffs, N.J.:
Prentice-Hall, 1967.

Gartner, A., and Riessman, F. *The Service Society and the Consumer Vanguard.* New York: Harper & Row, 1984.

Georgopoulos, B., and Mann, F. E. "The Hospital as an Organization." In J. S. Rakich and K. Darr (eds.), *Hospital Organization and Management.* New York: Wiley, 1978.

Gerson, E. "Rationalization and the Varieties of Technical Work." San Francisco: Tremont Research Institute, 1977. (Mimeographed.)

Gerson, E. *Memo on Human Information Systems.* San Francisco: Tremont Research Institute, July 16, 1981. (Mimeographed.)

Gerson, E., and Strauss, A. "Time for Living: Problems in Chronic Illness Care." *Social Policy,* 1975, *6,* 12–18.

Given, B., and Simon, S. "The Interdisciplinary Health Care Team." *Nursing Forum,* 1977, *26,* 165–184.

Glaser, B. G. *Theoretical Sensitivity.* Mill Valley, Calif.: Sociology Press, 1978.

Glaser, B. G., and Strauss, A. *Awareness of Dying.* Hawthorne, N.Y.: Aldine, 1965.

Glaser, B. G., and Strauss, A. *The Discovery of Grounded Theory.* Hawthorne, N.Y.: Aldine, 1967.

Glaser, B. G., and Strauss, A. *Time for Dying.* Hawthorne, N.Y.: Aldine, 1968.

Glaser, B. G., and Strauss, A. *Anguish.* Mill Valley, Calif.: Sociology Press, 1970.

Glaser, B. G., and Strauss, A. "Awareness Context of Social Interaction." *American Sociology Review,* 1974, *29,* 669–679.

Goffman, E. "Presentation of Self to Others." In *Presentation of Self in Everyday Life.* New York: Doubleday, 1959.

Goffman, E. *Behavior in Public Places.* New York: Free Press, 1963.

Goodykoontz, L. "Touch: Attitude and Practice." *Nursing Forum,* 1979, *18,* 4–16.

Gordon, G. "Nursing Diagnosis and the Diagnostic Process." *American Journal of Nursing,* 1976, *76* (8), 1298–1303.

Graham, N. "Done In, Fed Up, Burned Out!" *Journal of Emergency Medical Service,* Jan. 1981, pp. 14–29.

Gray, B. H. *Human Subjects in Medical Experimentation.* New York: Harper & Row, 1975.

Groff, B. "Dilemmas: Anatomy of a Malpractice Trial." *American Journal of Nursing,* 1985, *85* (3), 248–250.

Halberstam, M. S., and Lesher, S. *A Coronary Event.* New York: Popular Library, 1976.

Hamil, E. M. *People Power.* Publication no. 20-1623. Kansas City, Mo.: National League of Nursing, 1976.

Hastings Center Institute of Society, Ethics, and the Life Sciences. "Values, Ethics, and CBA in the Health Care." In *Implications of Cost Effective Analysis of Medical Technology*. Washington, D.C.: Office of Technology Assessment, 1980.

Hathaway, R. "The Swan-Ganz Catheter: A Preview." *Nursing Clinics of North America*, 1978, *13* (3), 389–497.

Herman, S. J. *Becoming Assertive: A Guide to Nurses*. New York: D. Van Nostrand, 1978.

Hilfiker, D. "Doctor's Mistake." *San Francisco Chronicle*, Sept. 16, 1984. (*This World*, pp. 7–9.)

Holloway, N. N. *Nursing and Critically Ill Adults*. Reading, Mass.: Addison-Wesley, 1979.

Housley, C. E. *Hospital Material Management*. Rockville, Md.: Aspen Corp., 1978.

Howard, J. "Humanization and Dehumanization of Health Care." In J. Howard and A. Strauss (eds.), *Humanizing Health Care*. New York: Wiley, 1975.

Howard, J., and Strauss, A. (eds.). *Humanizing Health Care*. New York: Wiley, 1975.

Huey, F. L. "What's on the Market? A Nurse's Guide." *American Journal of Nursing*, 1983, *83* (6), 902–910.

Hughes, E. C. *The Sociological Eye*. Hawthorne, N.Y.: Aldine, 1971.

Iglehart, J. K. "Another Chance for Technology Assessment." *New England Journal of Medicine*, 1983, *309,* 509–512.

Illich, I. *Medical Nemesis*. New York: Bantam Books, 1977.

Ingelfinger, F. J. "The Costs and Risks of a Diagnosis." *San Francisco Chronicle*, Oct. 28, 1978.

Ivancevich, R. E. "American Hospital Association Perspective: Legislation and Administrative Thrust in National Health Policy." In E. G. Jaco (ed.), *Evolving National Health Policy: Effects on Institutional Providers*. Proceedings of 1977 National Health Forum. San Antonio, Tex.: Trinity University Center for Professional Development in Health Administration, 1977.

Jacobs, K. D. "Does the Nurse Practitioner Involve the Patient in His Care?" *Nursing Outlook*, 1981, *28* (8), 501–505.

Jameton, A. *Nursing Practice: The Ethical Issue*. Englewood Cliffs, N.J.: Prentice-Hall, 1984.

Janowski, M. J. "Accidental Disconnections from Breathing Systems." *American Journal of Nursing,* 1984a, *84* (2), 241–244.

Janowski, M. J. "Feedback upon Ventilators." *American Journal of Nursing,* 1984b, *84* (12), 1494.

Jennett, B. *High Technology Medium Benefits and Burdens.* Oxford, England: Oxford University Press, 1986.

Jenny, J. "Patient Advocacy—Another Role for Nursing." *International Nursing Review,* 1979, *26* (6), 176–177.

Jobling, R. "Learning to Live with It: An Account of a Career of Chronic Dermatological Illness and Patienthood." In A. Davis and G. Horobin (eds.), *Medical Encounters.* London: Croom Helm, 1976.

Johnson, M. "Patients: Receivers or Participants?" In K. Barnard and K. Lee (eds.), *Promises, Patients and Politics: Conflicts in National Health Services.* London: Croom Helm, 1977.

Joint Commission on Accreditation of Hospitals. *Accreditation Manual for Hospitals.* Chicago: Joint Commission on Accreditation of Hospitals, 1984.

Jones, R. J. "The American Medical Association's Diagnostic and Therapeutic Technology Assessment (DATTA)." *Journal of American Medical Association,* 1983, *250,* 387–388.

Kalisch, B. "On Half Gods and Mortals: Aesculapian Authority." *Nursing Outlook,* 1975, *23* (1), 22–28.

Karch, F. E., and others. "Clinically Important Drug Interactions." *Nurses' Drug Alert,* 1979, *3* (Special Report), 25–40.

Kast, F. E., and Rosenzweig, J. E. "Hospital Administration and the Systems Concept." *Hospital Administration Quarterly,* 1966, *11,* 17–33.

Kennedy, J. *The Unmasking of Medicine.* London: Allen & Unwin, 1976.

King, I. M. *Toward a Theory of Nursing.* New York: Wiley, 1971.

King, L. S. "What Is a Diagnosis?" *Journal of the American Medical Association,* 1967, *202,* 714–718.

Knaus, W. A., Draper, E. A., Wagner, D., and Zimmerman, J. "An Evaluation of Outcome in Intensive Care." *Journal of Internal Medicine,* 1986, *104,* 410–418.

Knaus, W. A., Schroeder, S. A., and Davis, D. A. "The Impact of New Technology: The EMI Scanner." *Medical Care,* 1977, *15,* 533–542.

Kohnke, M. K. "The Nurse as Advocate." *American Journal of Nursing*, 1980, *81* (110), 2139.

Ladd, J. "Legalism and Medical Ethics." *Journal of Medicine and Philosophy*, 1979, *4* (11), 70–80.

Langford, T., and Prescott, P. A. "Hospitals and Supplemental Nursing Agencies: An Uneasy Balance." *Journal of Nursing Administration*, 1979, *11*, 16–20.

Leonard, J. "Legal Liabilities." In *Proceedings of AACN, 10th Annual Meeting*. Newport Beach, Calif.: American Clinical Association of Critical Care Nurses, 1983.

Levine, E. "Hospital Headlines." *Hospitals*, 1980, *54*, 18–19.

Levine, M. E. "The Ethics of Computer Technology of Health Care." *Nursing Forum*, 1980, *19* (2), 193–198.

Light, D. *Becoming a Psychiatrist.* New York: Norton, 1980.

Lofland, L. H. *The Craft of Dying: The Modern Face of Death.* Newbury Park, Calif.: Sage, 1978.

Longest, B. "Relationship Between Coordination Efficiency and Quality Care in General Hospitals." *Hospital Administration*, 1974, *19*, 65–86.

Lowin, A. "Participative Decision Making: A Model, Literature Critique, and Prescription for Research." *Organizational Behavior, Human Performance*, 1968, *3* (1), 68–106.

Lubkin, I. *Chronic Illness: Interventions for Health Professionals.* Belmont, Calif.: Wadsworth, 1986.

McBryde, C. M., and Blacklow, R. S. *Signs and Symptoms: Applied Pathological Physiology and Clinical Interpretation.* Philadelphia: Lippincott, 1970.

McConnell, E. A. *Burnout in the Nursing Profession: Coping Strategies, Causes and Costs.* St. Louis, Mo.: Mosby, 1982.

McDermott, W. "Evaluating the Physician and His Technology." *Daedalus*, 1977, *106*, 135–157.

McKinney, M. "The Newest Miracle Drug: Quality Circle in Hospitals." *Hospital and Health Services Administration*, 1984, *29*, 74–87.

Mann, K. W. *Deadline for Survival: A Survey of Moral Issues in Science and Medicine.* New York: Seabury Press, 1970.

Maslach, C. "Burned-Out." *Human Behavior*, 1976, *5* (9), 16–22.

Mitchell, W. E., Jr. "How to Deal with Poor Medical Care." *Journal of the American Medical Association*, 1976, *236*, 2875–2877.

Mizrath, T. "Managing Medical Mistakes: Ideology, Insularity and Accountability Among Internists-in-Training." *Social Science and Medicine,* 1984, *19* (2), 135–146.

Mockler, R. J. "Situational Theory of Management." *Harvard Business Review,* 1971, *49,* 146–148.

Monagle, J. F. "Risk Management Is Linked with Quality Care." *Hospitals,* 1980, *54* (17), 57–58.

Mundinger, M.O.N. "Primary Nurse—Role Evolution." *Nursing Outlook,* 1973, *21,* 643–645.

Murray, I. P. "Complications of Invasive Monitoring." *Medical Instrumentation,* 1981, *15* (2), 85–89.

Nagi, S. "Teamwork in Health Care in the U.S.: A Sociological Perspective." *Millbank Memorial Fund Quarterly: Health and Society,* 1975, *53,* 75–92.

National Academy of Sciences. *Assessing Quality of Health Care: An Evaluation.* Publication no. 76–04. Washington, D.C.: Institute of Medicine Publications, 1976.

Neuhauser, D. "The Hospital as a Matrix Organization." *Hospital Administration,* 1972, *17,* 8–25.

Nursing Development Conference Group. *Concept Formulation in Nursing: Process and Product.* Boston: Little, Brown, 1973.

Oberle, J. C. "Opinion Exchange: Was It Advocacy, Insubordination or Both?" *RN,* 1982, *45,* 109–113.

Office of Technology Assessment. *Development of Medical Technology: Opportunities for Assessment.* Washington, D.C.: U.S. Government Printing Office, Aug. 1976.

Office of Technology Assessment. *Assessing the Efficacy and Safety of Medical Technologies.* Washington, D.C.: U.S. Government Printing Office, 1978.

Olesen, V. L., and Whittaker, E. W. *The Silent Dialogue: A Study in the Social Psychology of Professional Socialization.* San Francisco: Jossey-Bass, 1968.

Orlikoff, J., and Snow, A. *Assessing Quality Circle in Health Care Settings.* New York: American Hospital Association Publications, 1984.

Partridge, K. B. "Nursing Values in a Changing Society." *Nursing Outlook,* 1978, *26,* 356–360.

Peplau, H. "Is Nursing's Self-Regulatory Power Being Eroded?" *American Journal of Nursing,* 1985, *85* (2), 140–143.

Perry, S. "The Brief Life of the National Center for Health Care Technology." *New England Journal of Medicine,* 1982, *307,* 1095-1100.

Petit, C. "The Debate on Ethic of Artificial Heart." *San Francisco Chronicle,* Sept. 19, 1985, p. 23.

Piazza, D., and Jackson, B. S. "Clinical Nurse Specialists: Issues, Power, and Freedom." *Supervising Nurse,* 1978, *9*(12), 47-51.

Pierpaoli, P. G. "Drug Therapy and Diet." *Drug Intelligence and Clinical Pharmacy,* 1972, *6,* 89-99.

Prescott, P. "Supplemental Nursing Service: Boon or Bane." *American Journal of Nursing,* 1979, *79* (12), 2140-2144.

Prescott, P. A. "Supplemental Nursing Service: How Much Do Hospitals Really Pay?" *American Journal of Nursing,* 1982, *82* (8), 1209-1213.

Regan, W. A. "How Do You Expose an Errant M.D.? . . . Very, Very Carefully." *RN,* 1978, *41* (5), 39-40.

Relman, A. S. "Assessment of Medical Practice: A Simple Proposal." *New England Journal of Medicine,* 1980a, *303,* 153-154.

Relman, A. S. "The New Medical-Industrial Complex." *New England Journal of Medicine,* 1980b, *303,* 963-970.

Relman, A. S. "An Institute of Health Care Evaluation." *New England Journal of Medicine,* 1982, *306,* 669-670.

Robinson, M. B. "Patient Advocacy and the Nurse: Is There a Conflict of Interest?" *Nursing Forum,* 1985, *22* (2), 58-63.

Rogers, M. A. *An Introduction to the Theoretical Bases for Nursing Practice.* Philadelphia: F. A. Davis, 1970.

"The Role of the Salesmen in Surgery." *San Francisco Chronicle,* May 24, 1978, p. AA1.

Roy, W. R. "Overutilization of Health Care." *Bulletin of the New York Academy of Medicine,* 1978, *54,* 132-138.

Russell, L. B. *Technology in Hospitals: Medical Advances and Their Diffusion.* Washington, D.C.: Brookings Institution, 1979.

Sang-O, R. "Organizational Determinants in Medical Quality: A Review of Literature." In R. C. Lake and J. Kreuger (eds.), *Organizational Change in Health Care Quality Assurance.* Rockville, Md.: Aspen Corp., 1984.

Schatzman, L, and Strauss, A. *Field Research.* Englewood Cliffs, N.J.: Prentice-Hall, 1973.

Schoenfeld, M. R. "Terror in ICU." *Forum on Medicine,* 1978, *1* (6), 4.

Schreiber, M., and others. "Vendor Use of Nurses in the Development of New Computer System." In H. G. Hefferman (ed.), *Fifth Annual Symposium on Computer Application in Medical Care, 1981, Washington, D.C.* New York: Institute of Electrical and Electronics Engineers, 1981.

Schroeder, R. E., Rhodes, A. M., and Shields, R. E. "Nurse Acuity Systems: Cash vs. Grasp." *Nursing Forum,* 1984, *21* (2), 72-77.

Schroeder, S. A. "Commentary: Why the Reservation About Medical Technology." *Proceedings of the Institute of Electrical and Electronics Engineers,* 1979, *9,* 1337-1339.

Schroeder, S. A., and Showstack, J. "The Dynamics of Medical Technology Use: Analyses and Policy Options." San Francisco: Institute for Health Policy Studies, School of Medicine, University of California, 1977.

Schroeder, S. A., Showstack, J. A., and Robert, H. E. "Frequency of Clinical Description of High-Cost Patients." *New England Journal of Medicine,* 1979, *300,* 1306-1309.

Selby, T. L. "Hospital RNs Feel Brunt of Budget Cuts." *American Nurse,* 1986, *18,* (1), 18-24.

Shepherd, M. D. *A Systems Approach to Hospital Medical Device Safety.* Outreach Series. Arlington, Va.: Association for the Advancement of Medical Instrumentation, 1983.

Shubin, S. "Burnout: The Professional Hazard You Face in Nursing." *Nursing,* 1978, *78* (7), 23-27.

Siegler, M., and Osmond, H. "Aesculapian Authority." *Hasting Center Studies,* 1973, *1* (2), 41-52.

Simborg, D. W. "DRG Creep: A New Hospital Acquired Disease." *New England Journal of Medicine,* 1981, *314,* 1602-1604.

Simms, L. M., and Lindbergh, J. B. *The Nurse Person.* New York: Harper & Row, 1979.

Simon, N. M. *The Psychological Aspects of Intensive Care Unit Nursing.* Bowie, Md.: John J. Brady, 1980.

Smith, C. S. "Outrageous or Outraged: A Nurse Advocacy Story." *Nursing Outlook,* 1980, *28* (10), 624-625.

Somer, A. R. *Hospital Regulations: The Dilemma of Public Policy.*

Princeton, N.J.: Industrial Relations Section, Princeton University, 1969.

Stacey, M. (ed.). "The Health Service Consumer: A Sociological Misconception." In *Sociology of National Health Services, Sociological Review Monograph #22.* London: Keele, 1976.

Starr, P. *The Social Transformation of American Medicine.* New York: Basic Books, 1982.

Steel, K., Gertman, P. M., Crescenzi, C., and Anderson, J. "Iatrogenic Illness on a General Medical Service at a University Hospital." *New England Journal of Medicine,* 1981, *304* (11), 638–641.

Stelling, J., and Bucher, R. "Vocabularies of Realism in Professional Socialization." *Social Science and Medicine,* 1973, *7,* 661–675.

Stepter, N. G. "Hospitalized Patients Work!" *Supervisor Nurse,* 1981, *12,* 55.

Stinson, R., and Stinson, P. "On the Death of a Baby." *Atlantic Monthly,* 1979, *244* (1), 64–72.

Storlie, F. J. "Burnout: The Elaboration of a Concept." *American Journal of Nursing,* 1979, *79* (12), 2105–2111.

Strauss, A. "Discovering New Theory from Previous Theory." In T. Shibutani (ed.), *Human Nature and Collective Behavior: Papers in Honor of Herbert Blumer.* Englewood Cliffs, N.J.: Prentice-Hall, 1970.

Strauss, A. *Chronic Illness and the Quality of Life.* St. Louis, Mo.: Mosby, 1975.

Strauss, A. *Negotiations: Varieties, Contexts, Processes, and Social Order.* San Francisco: Jossey-Bass, 1978.

Strauss, A. "Interorganizational Negotiation." *Urban Life,* 1982, *11* (3), 350–367.

Strauss, A. *Qualitative Analysis for Social Scientists.* New York: Cambridge University Press, 1986.

Strauss, A., and others. *Chronic Illness and the Quality of Life.* (2nd ed.) St. Louis, Mo.: Mosby, 1984.

Strauss, A. L., Fagerhaugh, S., Suczek, B., and Wiener, C. "Patients' Work in the Technologized Hospital." *Nursing Outlook,* 1981, *29,* 404–412.

Strauss, A. L., Fagerhaugh, S., Suczek, B., and Wiener, C.

"The Work of Hospitalized Patients." *Social Science and Medicine,* 1982, *16,* 977–986.

Strauss, A., Fagerhaugh, S., Suczek, B., and Wiener, C. *The Social Organization of Medical Work.* Chicago: University of Chicago Press, 1985.

Taylor, K. M., and Kelner, M. "Informed Consent—The Physician's Perspective." *Social Science and Medicine,* 1987, *24* (2), 135–143.

Taylor, M. B. "The Effects of DRGs on Home Health Care." *Nursing Outlook,* 1985, *33* (6), 281–287.

Thomas, L. *The Living Cell.* New York: Bantam Books, 1974.

Thompson, J. D., and Driers, D. "DRGs and Nursing." *Nursing and Health Care,* 1985, *6* (8), 435–439.

Thompson, R. "Organizational Consideration." In N. Graham (ed.), *Quality Assurance in Hospitals.* Rockville, Md.: Aspen Corp., 1982.

Trandel-Korenchuk, D. M., and Trandel-Korenchuk, K. M. "Legal Forum: Malpractice and Preventive Risk Management." *Nursing Administration Quarterly,* 1983, *7* (3), 75–80.

Tuma, J. Letter to Editor. *Nursing Outlook,* 1977, *25,* p. 546.

U.S. Department of Health and Human Services. *Health in United States.* Washington, D.C.: U.S. Government Printing Office, 1980.

Vecchio, T. J. "I Am Dazzled by Dehumanized Medicine." *Medical Economics,* 1977, *54* (14), 85.

Waitzkin, W., and Waterman, B. *The Exploitation of Illness in Capitalist Society.* Indianapolis, Ind.: Bobbs-Merrill, 1974.

Warner, J. D., and Kolff, W. J. "Cost of Home Dialysis Versus Institutional Dialysis." *Journal of Dialysis,* 1977, *1,* 67–73.

Warner, K. E. "Effects of Hospital Cost Containment on the Development and the Use of Medical Technology." *Millbank Memorial Fund Quarterly: Health and Society,* 1978, *56* (2), 187–211.

Weinberg, H. "Effecting Change in Hospital Performance: Issues and Realities." In N. Graham (ed.), *Quality Assurance in Hospitals.* Rockville, Md.: Aspen Corp., 1982.

Weiss, S. J. "Language of Touch." *Nursing Research,* 1979, *28,* 76–80.

Wiener, C., Fagerhaugh, S., Strauss, A., and Suczek, B. "Trajectories, Biographies and the Evolving Medical Technology Scene: Labor and Delivery and the Intensive Care Nursery." *Sociology of Health and Illness,* 1979, *1,* 261–283.

Wiener, C., Fagerhaugh, S., Strauss, A., and Suczek, B. "Patient Power: Complex Issues Need Complex Answers." *Social Policy,* 1980, *11,* 30–39.

Wiener, C., Fagerhaugh, S., Strauss, A., and Suczek, B. "What Price Chronic Illness?: Debates over Cost, Equity, and Technology." *Society,* 1982, *19* (2), 22–30.

Willens, R. M. "A Solution to Equipment Malfunction in the Critical Care Areas." In *Proceedings of the 17th AAMI Annual Meeting.* Arlington, Va.: Association for the Advancement of Medical Instrumentation, 1982.

Woodrow, M., and Bell, J. "Clinical Specialization: Conflict Between Reality and Theory." *Journal of Nursing Administration,* 1971, *1,* 23–28.

Wyers, M., Grove, S. K., and Pastorino, C. "Clinical Nurse Specialist: In Search for a Right Role." *Nursing and Health Care,* 1985, *6* (4), 203–207.

Zechhauser, R., and Stokey, E. *A Primer for Policy Analysis.* New York: Norton, 1978.

Zemaitis, M. "The Development of Critical Care Nursing." In *Proceedings of the 17th AAMI Annual Meeting.* Arlington, Va.: Association for the Advancement of Medical Instrumentation, 1982.

Zussman, J. "Think Twice About Becoming a Patient Advocate." *Nursing Life,* 1982, *6,* 46–50.

Index

247